Early Diagnosis and Therapy in Cerebral Palsy

PEDIATRIC HABILITATION

series editor   ALFRED L. SCHERZER

Cornell University Medical Center
New York, New York

Early Diagnosis and Therapy in Cerebral Palsy

A Primer on Infant Developmental Problems
Second Edition, Revised and Expanded

Alfred L. Scherzer
The New York Hospital-Cornell Medical Center
New York, New York

Ingrid Tscharnuter
New York University
New York, New York

MARCEL DEKKER, INC.   New York and Basel

Library of Congress Cataloging-in-Publication Data

Scherzer, Alfred L.
  Early diagnosis and therapy in cerebral palsy : a primer on infant
developmental problems / Alfred L. Scherzer, Ingrid Tscharnuter. --
2nd ed., rev. and expanded.
      p.   cm. -- (Pediatric habilitation ; vol. 6)
  Includes bibliographical references.
  ISBN 0-8247-8109-0 (alk. paper)
    1. Cerebral palsied children.   I. Tscharnuter, Ingrid.
II. Title. III. Series: Pediatric habilitation ; v. 6.
  [DNLM: 1. Cerebral Palsy--diagnosis. 2. Cerebral Palsy--therapy.
3. Child Development.   W1 PE167K v. 6 / WS 342 S326e]
RJ496.C4S344   1990
618.92'836--dc20
DNLM/DLC
for Library of Congress   89-25866
                                                                CIP

MARCEL DEKKER, INC.
270 Madison Avenue, New York, New York 10016

Current printing (last digit):
10 9 8 7 6 5 4 3 2

PRINTED IN THE UNITED STATES OF AMERICA

*To the many children and their families
from whom we have learned so much, and
who have enabled us to share with others*

Preface to the Second Edition

The first edition of *Early Diagnosis and Therapy in Cerebral Palsy*, issued in 1982, sought to fill a major need for professionals in bringing together in one source comprehensive information regarding diagnosis and management of the very young child with cerebral palsy. At the same time, we hoped to demonstrate how this framework might serve equally in developing programs for other types of nonprogressive deficits with similar needs. That we succeeded in filling this gap is well illustrated by the wide use of this text over the years and its continued demand by a variety of professionals.

In the years since the original issue, there have been many new and exciting developments in the field. Among these of major interest are new approaches to early screening and identification, refinements in concepts and approaches to therapy, considerations of alternative surgical approaches to treatment, and an explosion in early intervention strategies increasingly based more on an educational than on a traditional medical model.

Clearly the time has come to incorporate these developments into this text which has found much favor with our colleagues. We therefore take pleasure in bringing forth this second edition with the hope that it will continue to fill the needs of those devoted to the care of the handicapped child in this ever-changing field.

Alfred L. Scherzer
Ingrid Tscharnuter

Preface to the First Edition

Until relatively recent years, cerebral palsy was primarily of professional interest to a limited number of specialists dealing with specific aspects of treatment, such as orthopedics and neurology. Indeed, these are the specialities which initially shaped its definition and scope, dating from the days of Little and Freud. Children came to attention late, when significant limitations in development and milestones were noted, or severe orthopedic deficits were apparent. Intervention was frequently concerned with static neurologic assessment, and treatment often exclusively focused upon orthopedic surgery or a form of limited individual muscle therapy. The approach was to deal with the specific functional deficits as they appeared.

A much broader concept has subsequently emerged with the awareness that cerebral palsy represents a major multidisciplinary developmental disorder in which timely intervention by a variety of specialties is essential, and a coordinated, directed approach is required. In addition, traditional therapy involving individual muscle training has given way—mostly through clinical work with cerebral palsy—to a more comprehensive and dynamic approach of movement education which emphasizes the sensorimotor duality and is therefore conducive to learning new motor skills. Clinical experience with cerebral palsy has also promoted an expansion in the understanding of sensorimotor development. Today, abnormal motor behavior typically associated with cerebral palsy is seen as the outcome of a long process of postural compensations to underlying deficits, such as abnormal postural tonus or poor integration of postural reflexes. While early and primary postural compensations consist of more subtle deviations from the norm, motor skills building on these deviant patterns become more and more abnormal.

Newer knowledge concerning infant development and recognition of early common findings among infants with nonprogressive central nervous system deficits has now placed cerebral palsy within the spectrum of major developmental disabilities. In fact, its early identification and management presently serve as a model for other types of multiply handicapping conditions.

Recent perinatal management and neonatal intensive care technologies have further influenced the outlook for the child with potential disability. Children are now surviving who until recently had an abysmal prognosis. Evidence indicates a reduction, as well, in degree of disability, although an increase in severity is suggested especially among those high-risk and low-birth-weight infants who formerly did not survive. It seems likely that chronic developmental disorders in children are destined to be a major and increasing concern for pediatrics of the future.

It is in this setting that the concepts of early diagnosis and intervention have taken root and a sizable literature has emerged. Current data are clinically supportive of early intervention and the notion is intuitively appealing on the basis of developmental theory. An explosive interest has been generated in this field, yet there is a paucity of sources available for comprehensive reference and documentation.

The present text attempts to fill this gap by putting into perspective the evolution of cerebral palsy from a narrow focus as an orthopedic disability to a broadly conceived developmental disorder. The emphasis is on the process of developmental diagnosis, and current clinical approaches to evaluation, management, and treatment are detailed. The need for continuous, systematic, and standardized re-evaluation is stressed. Suggestions are made for developing research methods which will ultimately lead to establishing the effectiveness of any given treatment approach.

It is hoped that the text will provide a useful guide for those who deal with a wide variety of developmental disabilities in young children. Considerable emphasis is placed on identifying early patterns of postural maladjustments so that they can be corrected as far as possible before leading to more severe abnormalities. Its focus is to provide a more uniform and standardized approach to diagnosis and treatment. Only in this way will it be possible to objectively evaluate and guide individual therapy activities. Ultimately, this will greatly aid in the much needed quest for research methodologies and firm data concerning the early intervention process.

Alfred L. Scherzer
Ingrid Tscharnuter

Contents

1

Definition of Cerebral Palsy and Scope of the Problem

CEREBRAL PALSY IN HISTORICAL PERSPECTIVE

While the physician Cazauvielh was the first to study cerebral paralysis scientifically [1], it is a French orthopedic surgeon who is credited with expressing the earliest professional interest in cerebral palsy. Delpech's influence helped form the basis for treatment. Delpech was concerned with the deformities resulting from polio-myelitis. His description of the tendo achilles lengthening for equinus was the first published in the literature [2]. The procedure caught the interest of John Little, an English orthopedist, who himself had contracted polio that left a residual equinus deformity (Fig. 1). Little consulted Delpech about the operation, but was discouraged because of the possibility of complicating infection. Subsequently, Little went to Germany, where the procedure was also being developed, and underwent a successful operation performed by Dr. George Stromeyer.

Little was impressed with the theory and aims of the tendo achilles lengthening and upon his return to England incorporated it into his practice, and became quite adept at the procedure. He also took an increasing interest in correction of various deformities in children [3]. Among these conditions he began to recognize many associated with paralysis, and particularly with generalized spasticity [4]. His definitive work in 1861 drew upon 20 years of experience and documented possible correlations between abnormality of pregnancy, labor, delivery, and subsequent developmental deficit [5]. Little reasoned that spasticity and deformity were primarily due to cerebral hemor-

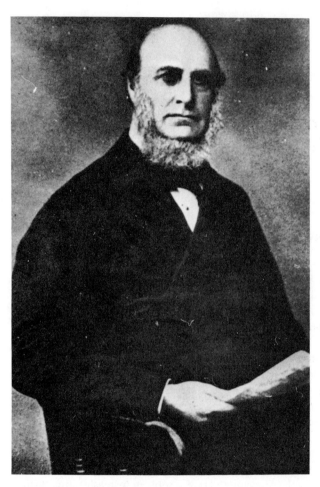

Figure 1 W. John Little, English orthopedist whose studies of cerebral palsy formed the basis of modern treatment.

rhage and anoxia secondary to trauma of the birth process (Fig. 2). Thus the entity known as Little's disease became established.

Interest in the condition spread to other medical disciplines. Gowers was among the earliest physicians to support Little's view [6]. Osler showed the neuroanatomical correlation of structural brain pathology and spastic paralysis [7].

Freud, initially practicing as a neurologist concerned with children, became greatly interested in the relationship of nonprogressive neurological deficits and prematurity [8]. He placed greater emphasis on intrauterine developmental abnormality and less on trauma than had Little (Fig. 3).

The interest in identification and etiology of spastic conditions initiated in the latter part of the nineteenth century maintained only limited momentum early into the twentieth century. Specific approaches to treatment were also slow in developing and had relatively little impact. Physical therapy made a start in the United States through the work of Jennie Colby at Children's Hospital in Boston [9]. Colby was a gymnast with an interest in massage therapy, which she channeled into developing remedial exercises for a variety of paralytic conditions. Her work was purely empirical and was incorporated into the program of the newly emerging neurology clinic established by Crothers. Here the new concepts of psychological aspects and mental health were added by Elizabeth Lord [10].

Orthopedic surgery to correct specific deformity gained greater popularity through the work of Stoffel. He perfected neurectomy as a specific procedure for managing contractures [11]. Surgery was viewed enthusiastically because of the easily measurable immediate and selected improvement. However, initial surgical benefit was often followed by disappointing long-term results.

As the psychological, developmental, neurological, and surgical considerations became more apparent, a broader approach was needed. The impetus began with Crothers and the interdisciplinary model in Boston, and was greatly expanded upon by Winthrop Phelps, an orthopedist who became devoted to finding ways to meet the needs of handicapped children, and who ultimately established a comprehensive community rehabilitation center in Maryland [12]. Phelps demonstrated the multispecialty approach in the period before world War II, when interest within the medical field was relatively scarce.

The years immediately following the war saw a merger of the extensive experience gained with rehabilitation medicine and rapid maturation in a variety of medical specialties. Renewed interest in the handicapped child

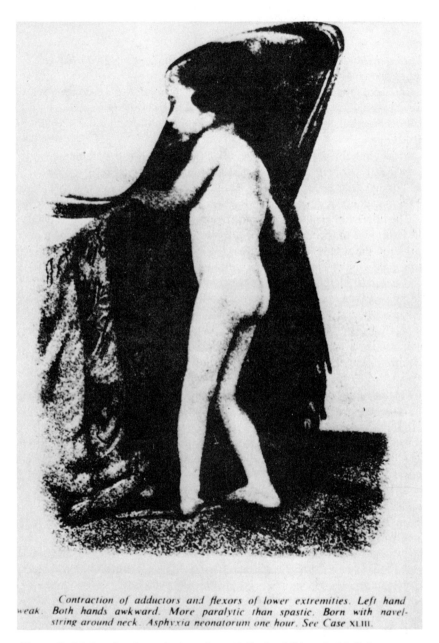

Contraction of adductors and flexors of lower extremities. Left hand weak. Both hands awkward. More paralytic than spastic. Born with navel-string around neck. Asphyxia neonatorum one hour. See Case XLIII.

Figure 2 Little related paralysis and spasticity in children to birth trauma (from Ref. 5).

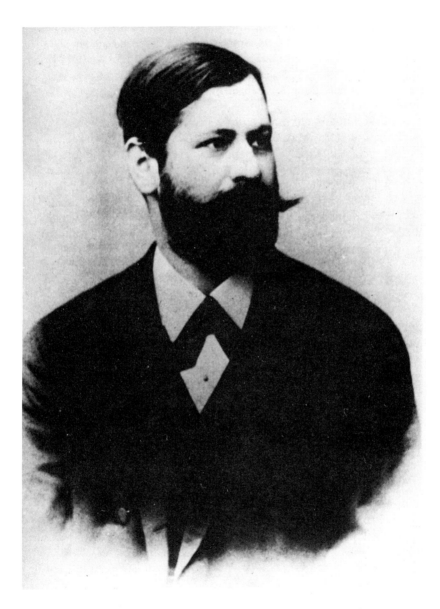

Figure 3 Sigmund Freud studied nonprogressive neurological deficits and prematurity in children.

became apparent in a number of professional groups. Community demands for action began to stir. The National Society for Crippled Children and Adults (Easter Seal Society) established a Cerebral Palsy Division in 1946 with a National Advisory Medical Council. This group of professionals soon recognized the need for a forum for interdisciplinary information and exchange of ideas.

It was in this setting that the Americal Academy for Cerebral Palsy (AACP) was born in Chicago in 1947 [13]. Conceived as a multispecialty professional organization to stimulate research and training in the field of the handicapped child, the AACP joined together the major medical disciplines with related therapy, educational, and psychological services. The founders, all of whom were in the original Easter Seal Group, had become convinced that only a combined effort could hope to have any measurable impact (Fig. 4). The founders of the Academy included Phelps, who was the first president, Temple Fay (neurophysiologist), Bronson Crothers (neurologist), Meyer Perlstein (pediatrician), George Deaver (physiatrist), and Earl Carlson (internist). What started as a small forum for discussion and interprofessional education was the beginning of a midcentury resurgence of interest and effort on behalf of the handicapped child [14].

Demand for local services and facilities was a simultaneous occurrence. A local chapter of the cerebral palsy committee was established in New York in 1948 [15]. Among its programs, it sponsored local hospital diagnostic services and provided treatment and educational programs based largely on the model developed in Maryland by Phelps in the 1930s. A New York State and finally a national United Cerebral Palsy Association followed with the subsequent development of more than 300 local chapters throughout the United States [16].

Of necessity, the emphasis of these programs was on diagnosis and treatment of the child with established deficits, frequently severe deformity of a long-standing nature. Children were being seen with degrees of deformity comparable to Little's reports of a century before. The difference lay in an approach much broader than orthopedics alone. In addition to the medical specialties, psychological services, and therapies, serious effort was made to provide appropriate special education, needed supportive social service, and family mental problems. As services developed and identification of the already handicapped became more efficient, there has been an increasing trend away from a rehabilitative to a "habilitative" approach. The aim is to employ whatever means necessary to bring a child to a level of maxi-

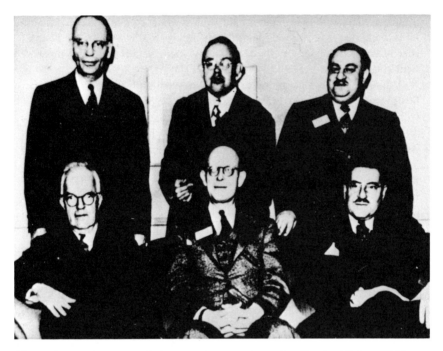

Figure 4   The founders of the American Academy for Cerebral Palsy, 1947. Standing (left to right). Dr. George Deaver (physiatrist), Dr. Earl Carlson (internist), Dr. Meyer Perlstein (pediatrician). Seated (left to right): Dr. Bronson Crothers (neurologist), Dr. Winthrop Phelps (orthopedist), Dr. Temple Fay (neurophysiologist).

mum potential in all areas of development, and particularly to ensure functional independence as an individual.

Technological developments in perinatal care from the late 1960s to the present have given further impetus to this concept. Improved obstetrical management of the high-risk mother complements a system of intensive neonatal care to reduce mortality significantly and selectively lower morbidity from neurological and developmental deficit [17]. A greater number of infants formerly classified as at risk, are living, and more effective methods of identifying neurological abnormality earlier enhance this trend. Contributions from the areas of developmental psychology and neurology, and experience of transdisciplinary methods with very young children have been particularly influential [18].

A parallel and logical outcome is early intervention treatment. Still imperfect in many respects, the present system of care has generally "caught up" with the late case of untreated and multiple deficit. In this respect, the goals of the 1950s to treat those with existing definitive handicaps are being met. As has been the case in the management of many medical conditions, the initial emphasis and interest lies with the most obvious and severe forms of the condition. As these become treated and greater understanding of cause is approached, emphasis is placed on more subtle forms and, finally, early diagnosis and treatment. So it is with cerebral palsy as we approach the turn of a new century. The data on the effect of early intervention are still emerging, but clearly are encouraging [19] (see Chap. 9).

In little more than 100 years, there has been a virtual revolution in concept and thought concerning cerebral palsy. Conceived initially as an orthopedic deficit with a neurological basis, it has come to be recognized as a multihandicapping condition requiring the attention of many specialties and services. But more than this, it is seen as a major disorder in development—a disability which emerges as the child grows—requiring early identification and management. Thus the orthopedic disease has become the prototype of the developmental disability and has facilitated a better understanding of the dynamics of developmental problems in children.

Recognition of this broader concept was given in 1977 when the AACP officially became the American Academy for Cerebral Palsy and Developmental Medicine (AACPDM) [20]. Little's early concern for the deformed child thus has merged at last with the broader area of the developmentally disabled.

TOWARD A DEFINITION OF CEREBRAL PALSY

Confusion continues to exist concerning the term cerebral palsy and its generally accepted meaning. Cerebral palsy refers to a *nonprogressive* central nervous system deficit. The lesion may be in a single or multiple locations of the brain, resulting in definite motor and possibly sensory abnormality. It occurs as a result of in utero factors, events at the time of labor and delivery (congenital cerebral palsy), or a variety of factors in the early developing years (acquired cerebral palsy). The former is estimated to account for 85% and the latter 15% of cases [21].

Burgess was the first to make use of the term in 1888 [22]. Soon after it appeared in the English literature by Osler [7] and Sachs and Peterson [23], in France by Brissaud [24], and among the influential Germans by Rosenberg [25] and Freud [26]. Phelps was the major popularizer in the United States. In conjunction with Phelps' work in developing a comprehensive treatment program, cerebral palsy came to be known as the major nonprogressive motor deficit occurring in children [27]. The AACPDM and the United Cerebral Palsy Associations have both reinforced the developmental aspects of the definition [28].

In addition to the motor deficit, other associated handicaps are frequently present. These include abnormalities of vision (25%) [29], hearing and speech (greater than 50%) [30], seizure disorders (one-third) [31], mental retardation (50-75% depending on motor severity) [32], learning disabilities among the vast majority, and frequent social, emotional, and interfamily problems. In every sense, therefore, the term conveys the concept of a multiply handicapping condition.

Confusion of terms and overlap with other nonprogressive central nervous system (CNS) disorders may be present. Cerebral palsy is a static *motor* deficit with associated handicaps. The primary *motor* nature of the condition provides a clear distinction from mental retardation syndromes, organic brain deficits, attention deficit disorder, autism, or emotional disorders.

CLASSIFICATION OF CEREBRAL PALSY MOTOR TYPES

The motor pattern type of cerebral palsy may take several forms. The spastic variety is most common and correlates with a fixed lesion in the motor portion of the cerebral cortex and pyramidal tract dysfunction. Athetosis or dystonia reflects involvement in the extrapyramidal pathways. Frequently there is intermittent tension of trunk or extremities and a variety of uninhibited movement patterns, which sometimes have been the basis for confusion in classification. Ataxia relates to a cerebellar lesion. Mixed types are also increasingly common. These may include combinations of spasticity with athetosis or ataxia. Rigidity suggests a severe decerebrate lesion.

The clinical neurological lesion has variable distribution. Table 1 lists some definitions in common use.

Severity must also be considered as a basis for description and guide for prognosis and treatment. A descriptive statement should at least indicate whether the involvement is mild, moderate, or severe.

Type, distribution, and severity are essential aspects of the cerebral palsy diagnosis. They give meaning and direction to treatment and management of

Table 1   Distribution of Cerebral Palsy Types

Location	Description
Monoplegia	One extremity
Hemiplegia	Upper and lower extremity on one side
Paraplegia	Both lowers
Quadriplegia	Equal involvement of uppers and lowers
Diplegia	Quadriplegia with mild upper involvement

the patient, and provide a more uniform understanding of the problem than simply referring to a static motor encephalopathy.

Classification and uniformity of diagnostic description has always been controversial. Rosenberg was the first to tackle the problem [25]. He included categories of: generalized rigidity, paraplegic rigidity, bilateral spastic hemiplegia, bilateral athetosis, chorioform diplegia, and atypical forms.

Freud and Rie [16] made a slight refinement, giving more recognition to athetosis. Categories included spastic hemiplegia, generalized rigidity, paraplegic rigidity, paraplegic paralysis, double hemiplegia, generalized chorea, and bilateral athetosis.

These were the only classifications available until the mid-twentieth century and were largely the basis for understanding and describing the lesions up to that time. The modern era in classification dates from the work of Fay in 1950 [33]. He greatly elaborated on various clinical aspects of the movement disorder, perhaps encumbering the system beyond practical use:

Spastic paralysis-cerebral Nonspastic paralysis; atonic type
Athetosis-midbrain Deafness; tension; nontension; hemiplegia; tremor;
   cerebral release, emotional release, head, neck, arm; shudder-type;
   rotary type, dystonia type, flail type
Tremors and rigidities-basal ganglia Parkinsonism types; decerebrate types
Ataxia cerebellar, kinesthetic
High spinal spastic-medulla
Mixed-diffuse

Phelps greatly refined these categories into a simpler and more practical clinical scheme [34]. He included: flaccid paralysis, spasticity, rigidity, tremor, athetosis, and ataxia. This system was much more workable and usable just at the time of resurgence of interest and community activity in the field.

Some further refinements were added by the clinicians Perlstein, Crothers, and Paine [35,36], which slightly expanded Phelps' approach. Their influence was strong in the subsequent classification prepared by Minear for the American Academy for Cerebral Palsy. In addition to motor types, distribution and degree of involvement as well as extent of treatment required were included for the first time [37].

Physiological (Motor)
    Spasticity
    Athetosis Tension; nontension, dystonia, tremor
    Rigidity
    Ataxia
    Tremor
    Atonia (rare)
    Mixed
    Unclassified
Distribution
Severity
Treatment

Some ambiguity exists in several of the Minear motor types, for example, the distinction between tremor athetosis and a separate tremor category. How does tremor differ from ataxia? Is there a physiological equivalent of atonia, or is this part of a developmental stage from which one of the other types ultimately emerges? Are some motor patterns unclassfiable again because they represent transient developmental features only?

The relevancy of these questions becomes apparent when we consider the Minear classification was prepared at a time when cerebral palsy was diagnosed late and solely on the recognition of a fixed motor deficit type. The developmental characteristics of the condition, and especially the emerging nature of the neurological lesion, were not then well appreciated. Depending upon the age at which a child was initially seen, the motor features would be variably evident. A modern classification therefore must consider the early signs of developmental abnormality and the emerging motor type. Such a classification could dispel confusion regarding diagnosis and provide better communication among the various professionals dealing with the child. An attempt is made to develop this approach in Chapter 2.

ETIOLOGICAL CONSIDERATIONS

Congenital Cerebral Palsy

This refers to conditions in which the etiology is traced to intrauterine, natal, or perinatal factors and was estimated by Perlstein to include some 85% of all cases [21]. The complexity of etiological association to the condition itself and to various motor types was apparent even to Little. He recognized for example, that spastic paraplegia or diplegia was generally associated with a preterm but normal delivery, whereas spastic quadriplegia was more often found with an abnormal term delivery [5]. The major considerations are discussed below.

Maternal and Environmental Factors

Regardless of gestational age or birth weight, the maternal prenatal condition may have a significant effect on subsequent CNS development and pathology of the fetus. General health status and untreated medical conditions may be relevant. Effects of drugs, alcohol, tobacco, exposure to radiation, or environmental pollutants are all known to have some bearing on fetal development but the possible relation to cerebral palsy specifically is not established. Factors directly affecting maturation of the placenta are not clear but could be highly relevant. Maternal infection remains a major source of fetal CNS pathology. The primary conditions of concern are congenital rubella, toxoplasmosis, cytomegalovirus, and herpes. Each may be without serious or even noticeable clinical manifestations during gestation. The latest on the list of possible congenital infections is the acquired immune deficiency syndrome (AIDS). It is well established that in the case of AIDS spread through intrapartum contact there is a very significant frequency of severe developmental disorders, including primary CNS motor conditions consistent with cerebral palsy [38].

Prematurity

That prematurity is a major associated factor in cerebral palsy has been well established and is noted in at least a third of cases [39-47]. The multivariate nature of prematurity however, raises serious questions about discrete causal factors and many uncertainties remain unresolved.

Gestational age itself must be considered in addition to birth weight. The small-for-gestational-age (SGA) child appears less likely to have cerebral palsy and more at risk for genetic disorders, mental retardation, and global neurological deficit than the child who is of appropriate weight for gestational age (AGA) [48].

The role of neonatal asphyxia remains controversial among premature births, in spite of frequent incidence of respiratory distress syndrome and apnea in this group. Churchill [41], and Davies and Tizard [44], for example, found no greater percentage with asphyxia among children weighing less than 2000 g compared with controls. This is further confirmed by more recent studies from Australia of an entire cerebral palsy population cohort. Intrapartum asphyxia was not found to be a likely causative factor [49].

Intracranial hemorrhage, especially among premature babies is well established and has been related to rupture of a disproportionately large middle cerebral artery. This is given further support in the collaborative cerebral palsy study indicating significant anemia among affected premature babies as the only feature distinguishing them from nonaffected controls [50]. Intraventricular hemorrhage is associated particularly with very, very low-birth-weight infants, generally those weighing less than 1000 g and possibly below 500 g. The correlation with ventricular dilatation is particularly likely to be seen in the child who develops cerebral palsy.

Other aspects suggesting a relation especially to prematurity include intrauterine malnutrition [51] and intrinsic developmental disability of the fetus [52]. Disproportionate central nervous system maturation among prematures has also been suggested [53]. The issue of pre-existing or simultaneous congenital CNS anomalous development rather than a simple causal relationship to prematurity or asphyxia has been re-emphasized by Nelson and Ellenberg in analysis of the National Collaborative Study [54].

Perinatal Events

Neonatal asphyxia has been considered a most significant perinatal event. This may be related to obstetrical accident, dystocia, anesthesia, nuchal cord or other mechanical problems, or intrinsic pulmonary deficit of the infant [55]. However, the recent work of Nelson [56] and Blair and Stanley [49] suggests that such intrapartum events as asphyxia may well be less of a contributory cause than has been traditionally thought. This is further confirmed by the work of Freeman and Nelson [57]. Intracranial hemorrhage appears to be a less likely causative event at birth for the full-term child. Infection during the perinatal period may be significant, particularly if it leads to sepsis or meningitis. Hyperbilirubinemia of the newborn due to Rh factor, ABO, or other blood group incompatability was formerly a major factor in development of kernicterus, milder forms of athetosis, or mixed forms of cerebral palsy. Its impact has been greatly reduced by improved methods of early identification, better exchange transfusions, and above all, the preventive use of anti-Rh (D) γ globulin to immunize the prospective mother immediately after her first pregnancy [58]. Neonatal jaundice due to sepsis or physiological immaturity of the liver may still require careful attention.

Primary Congenital Anomalies

Malformations of the CNS may be apparent at birth. Among those that may have a bearing on a fixed motor lesions are hydrocephalus, anencephaly, encephalocele, and a variety of intracranial structural deficits, such as Sturge-Weber syndrome, neurofibromatosis, and other phakomatoses. The extent to which these are remediable when detected early would determine whether permanent residual CNS abnormality exists.

Acquired Cerebral Palsy

Data regarding the incidence of fixed intracranial lesions with permanent residua which develop beyond the perinatal period are limited. Records of Perlstein's cases suggest approximately 15% [21], although studies of such lesions in the general population suggest an astonishingly higher frequency [59]. The major categories include CNS infections, intracranial hemorrhage due to primary vascular accident, or secondary to a thrombosis from a cardiac lesion, or sickle cell anemia.

Late onset or inadequately treated hydrocephalus may be a major factor. Trauma is particularly common once the child begins to walk and develops independence in the preschool period. Neoplastic intracranial lesions are not rare in the early developing years and may be associated with permanent residua [60].

Genetic Cerebral Palsy

A possible hereditary basis for cerebral palsy has been of considerable historic interest and concern. Examples of multiple cases within a given family lend credence to an earlier popular notion suggesting this possibility. However, objective review generally substantiates a pregnancy or birth history which could explain multiple involvement. Nevertheless, there are well-documented cases of apparent genetically determined lesions of spastic paraplegia, generalized athetosis, and ataxia [61]. A pattern of autosomal dominance is generally seen and may be traceable through several generations. Pathology in the case of spastic paraplegia is a structural deficit in the pyramidal tract in the upper cervical area [62].

Trends in Epidemiology

Incidence and Prevalence

From the time of John Little, until the resurgence of interest in the middle of this century, information about the extent of cerebral palsy has been limited. The first major study was conducted in the area around Schenectady, New York, in 1949 [63]. Phelps' research followed shortly thereafter and used an estimated prevalence figure of 7 per 100,000 population for all ages [64]. This was an often quoted statistic and difficult to compare with other studies covering children up to age 21 years [65]. Comparison can best be made with incidence data. Perlstein's figure of 7 per 1000 live births has been a well-accepted standard [66]. The subsequent studies of Hagberg et al. [67] and Franco and Andrews indicated a reduction in case incidence of nearly two-thirds through the 1970s [68]. More recent data of Paneth and Kiely suggest a figure of 2 per 1000 live births both for the United States and overall world incidence [69]. Also, possible increased severity must be strongly considered [70-71].

Factors affecting this trend include improved obstetrical management [72] and the technological success of increasingly sophisticated perinatal centers [73], especially in caring for premature infants weighing less than 1500 g [74], and without severe respiratory problems or intracranial hemorrhage [75]. Reduction in frequency and improved management of maternal infection, particularly rubella, is also significant.

Cerebral Palsy Types and Distribution

Considerable change is also noted in relative frequency of the major cerebral palsy motor types. Spasticity continues to be most common and is generally considered to be present in greater than 50% of cases [68]. A considerable reduction is noted now in spastic diplegia (generally associated with prematurity), especially among infants weighing more than 1000 g at birth. Interestingly, little change is noted now in frequency of spastic quadriplegia [67]. Athetosis was formerly noted in one-third of cases, and has been reduced to 10% or less [68], largely as a result of both preventive measures and/or treatment of neonatal hyperbilirubinemia.

Ataxia due to a fixed cerebellar lesion is seen in 5-10% of cases, and appears to be unchanged. Rigidity was thought to comprise about 1% of cases

[21]. Current clinical experience suggests this to be a rarely used category. This may reflect a better understanding of developmental neurological deficit; many cases formerly falling into this category are now more appropriately classified as athetosis with tension or mixed forms.

Mixed types of cerebral palsy also appear to be more commonly identified than previously, and are now probably only second in importance to spasticity. The opportunity for early initial and subsequent long-term observation seems to favor this category increasingly and may give a more accurate picture of the diffuse involvement which can be identified as the central nervous system matures.

Degree of Severity

About a third of patients have generally been considered to be equally distributed among the mild, moderate, and severely involved categories. A review by Franco and Andrews, however, has indicated (Table 2) considerable differences between premture and full-term infants [68].

The greater degee of profound involvement among premature babies is of significance since this remains a major etiologic category. Indeed, the improvement in survival of low and very low-birth-weight infants appears to suggest an increase in both incidence of cerebral palsy as well as greater severity of the condition among those affected infants in this weight category [75,76].

Associated Handicaps

No current studies include specific data on extent of visual, speech, and hearing deficits, seizure disorders, or mental retardation in association with cerebral palsy. However, some inferences can be made using knowledge

Table 2   Degree of Severity of Cerebral Palsy

Degree of Severity	Prematures (%)	Full-Term (%)
Profound	33	20
Moderate	27	36
Slight	40	44

Source: From Ref. 64.

about current trends in the condition. Less high-frequency hearing loss is probably found since this was seen regularly in athetosis. Both seizure disorders and degree of mental retardation closely parallel motor severity of cerebral palsy, and will reflect the pattern of greater involvement among very small premature infants. A greater recognition of associated severe perceptual-motor and other learning disabilities is now evident.

CURRENT TRENDS

The apparent considerable reduction in overall incidence of cerebral palsy has recently come under critical review [76]. It appears to be selective for those upper birth-weight infants formerly subject to abnormal events in the immediate perinatal period. Here there has been a dramatic effect in reduction of morbidity relating to developmental deficits, in association with improved obstetrical and perinatal care. Low-birth-weight prematures, on the other hand, are now surviving in increasing numbers and may well be subject to severe developmental risk [77]. Data from Sweden indicating a persistently high frequency of spastic quadriplegia in spite of reduced cerebral palsy incidence support this concept [67]. Current progress in maternal and infant care indeed confirms greater survival of "at-risk" children. Moreover, survival of those subject to greatest physiological stress is more likely to be associated with definite neurological deficit in the form of cerebral palsy [69].

In contrast with Little's day, we are fortunate in now having available the techniques for early identification and tools for early intervention which may enable survivors, even those with severe involvement, to develop some independent function and eventually make their contribution to society. This has become possible as the early limited orthopedic approach has increasingly expanded to include multiple professionals, all of whom must deal with the array of needs of the developmentally disabled child.

REFERENCES

1. Cazauvielh, J. Recherches sur l'agenesie cerebral et la paralysie congeniale. *Arch Gen Med.* 1827.

2. Delpech, M. Tenotomie de tendon d'Achilles, in Churgerie Clinique de Montpellier, Observations et Reflexions Tirees des Travaux de Chirurgie Clinique de Cette Ecole. Paris, Gabon, 1828, p. 181.

3. Little, W. Course of lectures on deformation of the human frame. Lecture number VIII. *Lancet* i:318, 1843.

4. Little W. *On the Nature and Treatment of the Deformities of the Human Frame.* London, Longman, Brown, Green and Longman, 1853.

5. Little W. On the influence of abnormal parturition, difficult labours, premature birth, and asphyxia neonatorum on the mental and physical condition of the child, especially in relation to deformities. *Trans. Obstet. Soc. London*, 3:293, 1861.

6. Gowers, W. On birth palsies. *Lancet* i:709, 1888.

7. Osler, W. The Cerebral Palsies of Children: A Clinical Study from the Infirmary for Nervous Diseases. Philadelphia, Blakiston, 1889.

8. Freud, S. Die infantile cerebrallahmung in Nothnagel, J.: Specialle Pathologie und Therapie, Band IX, Th.III. Vienna, Holder, 1897.

9. Colby, J. Massage and remedial exercises in the treatment of children's paralysis: Their difficulties in use. *Boston Med. Surg. J.* 173:696, 1915.

10. Lord, E. Children Handicapped by Cerebral Palsy. New York, Commonwealth Fund, 1937.

11. Stoffel, A. The treatment of spastic contracture. *Am. J. Orthop. Surg.*, 10:611, 1913.

12. Phelps, W. The treatment of cerebral palsies. *J. Bone Joint Surg.* 22: 1004, 1940.

13. Wolf, J. The Results of Treatment in Cerebral Palsy. Springfield, Charles C. Thomas, 1969, pp. 10-11.

14. Vining, E., Accardo, P., Rubenstein, J., Farrell, S., and Roizen, N. Cerebral palsy: a pediatric developmentalist's overview. *Am. J. Dis. Child.* 130:643, 1976.

15. Katz, A. Parents of the Handicapped. Springfield, Charles C. Thomas, 1961, p. 23.

16. United Cerebral Palsy. The Story of U.C.P. New York, 1949.

17. Merkatz, I., and Johnson, K. Regionalization of perinatal care for the United States. *Clin. Perinatol.* 3:271, 1976.

18. Haynes, U. The First Three Years—Programming for Atypical Infants and Their Families. New York, United Cerebral Palsy Association, 1974.

19. Tjossem, T. D. (Ed.). Intervention Strategies for the High Risk Infant. Baltimore, University Park Press, 1976.

20. Greenspan, L. The conception, growth, and development of the developmentalist. Presidential address. American Academy for Cerebral Palsy and Developmental Medicine, Atlanta, 1977.

21. Perlstein, M. Infantile cerebral palsy: classification and clinical observations. *JAMA* 149:30, 1952.

22. Burgess, D. A case of cerebral birth palsy. *Med. Chron. Manchester*, 9: 471, 1888.

23. Sachs, B., and Peterson, F. A study of cerebral palsies in early life-based upon an analysis of one hundred and forty cases. *J. Nerv. Ment. Dis.* 17:295, 1890.

24. Brissaud, E. Maladie de Little et tabes spasmodique. *Sem. Med.* 14:89, 1894.

25. Rosenberg, L. Der cerebralen Kinderlähmungen Kassowitz. *Beitr. Kinderheilkd.* Neue Folge IV, 1893.

26. Freud, S., and Rie, C. Klinische Studien Uber Die Hoslbseitige Cerebral-Lähmung der Kinder, Vienna, Perles, 1891.

27. Phelps, W. Let's define cerebral palsy. *Crippled Child* 16:4, 1948.

28. O'Reilly, D. History of the American Academy for Cerebral Palsy and Developmental Medicine. Washington, D.C. AACPDM, 1979.

29. Breakey, A. Ocular findings in cerebral palsy. *Arch. Ophthalmol.* 53: 852, 1955.

30. Vernon, M. Clinical phenomena of cerebral palsy and deafness. *Except. Child.* 36:743, 1970.

31. Robinson, R. The frequency of other handicaps in children with cerebral palsy. *Dev. Med. Child. Neurol.* 15:305, 1973.

32. Hopkins, T., Bice, H., and Colton, K. Evaluation and Education of the Cerebral Palsy Child. Washington, D.C., Intl. Council for Exceptional Children, 1954.

33. Fay, T. Cerebral palsy: medical considerations and classification. *Am. J. Psychiatry* 107:180, 1950.

34. Phelps, W. Etiology and diagnostic classification of cerebral palsy. In, Proceedings of the Cerebral Palsy Institute. New York, Association for the Aid of Crippled Children, 1950.

35. Perlstein, M. Medical aspects of cerebral palsy. *Nervous Child* 8:128, 1949.

36. Crothers, B., and Paine, R. The Natural History of Cerebral Palsy. Cambridge, Harvard University Press, 1959.

37. Minear, W. A classification of cerebral palsy. *Pediatrics* 18:841, 1956.

38. Rubinstein, A. Pediatric AIDS. *Curr. Probl. Pediatr.* 16:361, 1986.

39. Bandera, E., and Churchill, J. Prematurity and neurological disorders. *Henry Ford Hosp. Bull.* 9:414, 1961.

40. Berenberg, W. and Ong, B. Cerebral spastic paraplegia and prematurity. *Pediatrics* 33:496, 1964.

41. Churchill, J. The relationship of Little's disease to premature birth. *Am. J. Dis. Child.* 96:32, 1958.

42. Childs, B., and Evans, P. Birth weights of children with cerebral palsy. *Lancet* i:642, 1954.

43. Drillien, C. Growth and development in a group of children of very low birth weight. *Arch. Dis. Child.* 33:10, 1958.

44. Davies, P., and Tizard, J. Very low birth weight and subsequent neurological defect. *Dev. Med. Child. Neurol.* 17:3, 1975.

45. Eastman, N., Kohl, S., Maisel, J., and Kavaler, F. The obstetrical background of 753 cases of cerebral palsy. *Obstet. Gynecol. Surv.* 17:459, 1962.

46. McDonald, A. Cerebral palsy in children of very low birth weight. *Arch. Dis. Child.* 38:579, 1963.

47. Wright, F., Blough, R., Chamberlin, A., Ernest, T., Halstead, W., Meier, P., Moore, R., Naunton, R., and Newell, F. A controlled follow up study of small prematures born from 1952 through 1956. *Am. J. Dis. Child.* 124:506, 1972.

48. Scherzer, A., and Mike, V. Cerebral palsy and the low birth weight child. *Am. J. Dis. Child.* 128:199, 1974.

49. Blair, E., and Stanley, F. Intrapartum asphyxia: a rare cause of cerebral palsy. *J. Pediatr.* 112:515, 1988.

50. Churchill, J., Masland, R., Nagler, A., and Ashworth, M. The Etiology of Cerebral Palsy in Prematures. American Academy for Cerebral Palsy, New York, 1971.

51. Sabel, K., Olegard, R., and Victoria, L. Remaining sequelae with modern perinatal care. *Pediatrics* 57:652, 1976.

52. Polani, P. Prematurity and cerebral palsy. *Br. Med. J.* 2:1497, 1958.

53. Churchill, J. The relationship of Little's disease to premature birth. *Am. J. Dis. Child.* 96:32, 1958.

54. Nelson, K., and Ellenberg, J. Antecedents of cerebral palsy: multivariate analysis of risk. *New Engl. J. Med.* 315:81, 1986.

55. Roboz, P. Etiology of congenital cerebral palsy. *Arch. Pediat.* 79:233, 1962.

56. Nelson, K. What proportion of cerebral palsy is related to birth asphyxia? *J. Pediatr.* 112:572, 1988.

57. Freeman, J., and Nelson, K. Intrapartum asphyxia and cerebral palsy. *Pediatrics* 82:240, 1988.

58. Spellacy, W. (Ed.). Management of the High Risk Pregnancy. Baltimore, University Park Press, 1976.

59. Schoenberg, B. The spectrum of cerebrovascular disease in infants and children. Annual meeting, American Academy for Cerebral Palsy and Developmental Medicine. Atlanta, 1977.

60. Matson, D. Neurosurgery in Infancy and Childhood. Springfield, Charles C. Thomas, 1969.

61. Cooper, W., German, J., and Lame, E. Genetic implications of cerebral palsy. *J. Bone Joint Surg.* [Am.] 47:1673, 1965.

62. Silver, J. Familial spastic paraplegia with amyotrophy of the hands. *Ann. Hum. Genet.* 30:69, 1966.

63. Cruickshank, W., and Raus, G. Cerebral Palsy. Syracuse, Syracuse University Press, 1955.

64. Phelps, W. Etiology and diagnostic classification of cerebral palsy. In, Proceedings of the Cerebral Palsy Institute, New York, Association for the Aid of Crippled Children, 1950.

65. Henderson, J. Cerebral Palsy in Childhood. Edinburgh, Livingstone, 1961.

66. Perlstein, M., and Barnett, H. Nature and recognition of cerebral palsy in infancy. *JAMA* 148:1389, 1952.

67. Hagberg, B., Hagberg, G., and Olow, I. The changing panorama of cerebral palsy in Sweden 1954-1970. I. Analysis of general changes. *Acta Paediatr. Scand.* 64:187, 1975.

68. Franco, S., and Andrews, B. Reduction of cerebral palsy by neonatal intensive care. *Pediatr. Clin. North Am.* 24:639, 1977.

69. Paneth, N., Kiely, J., Stein, Z., and Susser, M. Cerebral palsy and newborn care. III. Estimated prevalence rates of cerebral palsy under differing rates of mortality and impairment of low-birth weight infants. *Dev. Med. Child. Neurol.* 23:801, 1981.

70. Nelson, K., and Ellenberg, J. Epidemiology of Cerebral Palsy. In Schoenberg, B. (Ed.): Advances in Neurology. Vol. 19. New York, Raven Press, 1978, pp. 421–435.

71. Kitchen, W., Rickards, A., Ryan, M., McDougall, A., Billson, F., Keir, E., and Naylor, F. A longitudinal study of very low-birth weight infants. II: results of controlled trial of intensive care and incidence of handicaps. *Dev. Med. Child. Neurol.* 21:582, 1979.

72. Fanaroff, A., and Merkatz, I. Modern obstetrical management of the low birth weight infant. *Clin. Perinatol.* 4:215, 1977.

73. Fitzhardinge, P., Kalman, E., Ashby, S., and Pape, K. Present status of the infant of very low birth weight treated in a referral neonatal intensive care unit in 1974. *Ciba Found. Symp.* 59:139, 1978.

74. Steward, A., and Reynolds, E. Improved prognosis for infants of very low birth weight. *Pediatrics* 54:724, 1974.

75. Steward, A., Turcan, D., Rawlings, G., Hart, S., and Gregory, S. Outcome for infants at high risk of major handicap. *Ciba Found. Symp.* 59:151, 1978.

76. Kiely, J., Paneth, N., Stein, Z., and Susser, M. Cerebral palsy and newborn care. I. Secular trends in cerebral palsy. *Dev. Med. Child. Neurol.* 23:533, 1981.

77. Kiely, J., Paneth, N., Stein, Z., and Susser, M. Cerebral palsy and newborn care. II. Mortality and neurological impairment in low-birth weight infants. *Dev. Med. Child. Neurol.* 23:650, 1981.

2

Developmental Evaluation and Differential Diagnosis

THE CONCEPT OF NORMAL NEUROLOGICAL MATURATION

The work of Gesell and others firmly established both uniformity and the concept of variation in the normal developmental sequence of children [1-3]. Acquaintance with this basic framework is essential to a working understanding on the growth process. More importantly, it is the cornerstone upon which identification and understanding of abnormal development rest. Some general principles of development are helpful in providing an overview.

There is a fairly orderly process from birth which is continuous with in utero development [4]. The neurophysiological basis of this process is generally considered to be ascending development of brain center control [5]. Initially, newborn infant behavior is largely of a reflex nature, mediated primarily through the brain stem. Maturation then proceeds toward "higher" centers, ultimately reaching independence in full voluntary control. Thus, one finds a progression in development in hierarchical levels of brain function. Also, it should be noted that some degree of voluntary movement is present even in the neonate. The infantile primitive reflexes then give way to more complex postural reflexes and proceed to full voluntary behavior. Also the initial mass behavior activity on a reflex basis is replaced by individual responses under voluntary control, and integration proceeds at the various levels of central nervous system (CNS) activity. Tone or the maintenance of the body in space, proceeds simultaneously as an integral part of the developmental process.

Motor maturation roughly proceeds in a cephalocaudal direction: motor control of the head, neck, and trunk preceding extension of the trunk, ultimate weight bearing, and walking.

Maturation of the normal central nervous system occurs simultaneously at many different levels. Although there is an orderly sequence in development, considerable variation is seen within a given child in achieving stages of motor and intellectual achievement. Thus, a child's intelligence may be considerably ahead of his or her locomotion ability, yet ultimately development may reach average levels. There is an acceptable degree of variation which exists among infants in reaching established levels of maturation.

Finally, motor development should be seen as a succession of integrated milestones leading to more complex and independent function [6]. Each stage is interdependent and relates closely to progressive control of higher centers of the nervous system and reduced influence of fixed reflex behavior [7]. Many stages will develop simultaneously. Each milestone, therefore, is not necessarily perfected before going on to the next [8]. Also, a "competition of motor patterns" is suggested in which a child carries out natural practicing of new activities with temporary suppression of others until learning is complete. Older and more established activities may then be resumed and added [9].

The challenge for those dealing with developmental problems in children is to accurately assess and comprehend the significance of delay which falls outside of the limits of variability. Is it normal or pathological? Knowledge of the normal, orderly sequence of developmental achievement, and patterns of integration of behavior is the basis upon which possibly significant deviation in maturation can be gauged. Appendix A includes a comprehensive outline of developmental stages and normal motor milestones for detailed reference, from ages two months to two years.

OVERVIEW OF ABNORMAL DEVELOPMENT

Although the theme of development is one of a continuum with many variations, its physiological basis is exceedingly complex and does not necessarily coincide with observable function at a given stage in the infant. Growth of nerve pathways, interconnections, and cell fiber proceeds actively to trunk and extremities while brain stem connections and influence remain predominant [10]. Myelination or development of the nerve insulation sheath, for example, is an active process thought, at least, to take up to the first two years before completion [11]. Thus the infant is initially dominated by the primitive reflexes mediated through the brain stem, and by mass response as physical and undoubtedly biochemical growth of the nervous system proceeds. The orderly process leads to gradual inhibition of initial primitive reflexes, emergence of postural reflex patterns, maturation of tone, and an increasing degree of voluntary behavior, simultaneously.

Malformation or insult to the central nervous system of the neonate will initially affect brain stem function. Alteration in appearance, intensity, or expression of primitive reflex behavior will result [12]. The normal course of early disappearance of primitive reflexes through inhibition pathways will be affected, with either delay or failure in the development of later postural reflex patterns [13].

Tone will be altered, either excessive or diminished quality will be present. This is mediated through brain stem pathways and will be an early indication of brain stem malfunction [14]. In particular, one may see a discrepancy between distal and proximal tone, that is, between the trunk and extremities.

Developmental milestones will be delayed in progression with prolonged fixation at a given stage. The degree of abnormality will relate to the degree of delay in brain stem inhibition and nerve pathway maturation. Both would be directly affected by the nature and degree of the central nervous system fixed pathology.

Motor abnormality of the total nervous system would appear relatively late in development of the infant as nerve pathways become more functional. This is a natural outcome of the selective nerve growth process. Differential rates or order of appearance of motor deficit are manifest. The abnormal motor patterns emerge as the damaged nervous system matures. For example, evidence of specific spasticity may be first noted only at 7 to 9 months of age. Athetosis will not generally be apparent before 18 months and may be delayed beyond two years. Ataxia is frequently not seen before 30 months to 3 years. Identification of mixed motor patterns may be further delayed, while the nervous system development progresses and relative dominance of one motor form interchanges with another.

The consequences of a fixed lesion of the central nervous system affecting the motor area and development must be seen as emerging and concomitant with growth of the system itself. It is a dynamic, active process, at least from the initial moment of postnatal life and probably earlier. Cerebral palsy is not to be conceived as one or more types of fixed motor disturbance but an array of developmental disorders which may affect the most primitive functions, and most sophisticated voluntary actions, and often both.

Particular focus should be on abnormal development in the child with a history of prematurity. Immature initial CNS development may result in

poor overall organizational ability which will ultimately need to be distinguished from true specific sensory and motor deficits. In fact, transient neurological deficits are common in such infants, and a long-term perspective on
progression in development is essential to achieve an accurate picture of developmental status.

Understanding of the broad developmental scope of the condition forms
the basis for both identification and intervention. It is no longer acceptable
to simply deal with the spastic foot, the athetoid posture, or the ataxic gait.
Consideration must be given as early as possible to definite recognition that
a global developmental abnormality exists, so that appropriate means can be
directed to remediate the spectrum of deficit of the entire nervous system.

PREDICTION OF DEVELOPMENTAL ABNORMALITY

Recognizing that early development is a dynamic and changing process has
led to extensive efforts of prediction of abnormality in young children. A
variety of developmental rating scales have bourgeoned within recent years,
with varying degrees of accuracy for prediction of (a) developmental delay,
(b) definite developmental abnormality, and (c) specific developmental diagnoses. Among those in use are the Prechtl [8], Amiel-Tison [15], Dubowitz
[16], Bayley [17], and Peabody [18] Scales, the Movement Assessment
Inventory (MAI) [19], and the Early Motor Pattern Profile (EMPP) [20].
Clearly, predictive power and sensitivity of any of these instruments varies
inversely with the age of the child. Moreover, none feature approaches to
early differential diagnosis considerations.

Irrespective of the use of, or findings from, various existing scales, it is
essential to have the perspective of a dynamic evaluative approach which (a)
identifies factors relating to significant risk for disability, and (b) utilizes
variables which can be followed to make an early determination of specific
developmental abnormality. The scales presently in use have limitations
in both these areas. With these considerations in mind, we offer, in the
following sections, a broad developmental evaluation approach to identification based upon clinical experience and long-term followup.

DEVELOPMENTAL EVALUATION APPROACH TO DIAGNOSIS

The complex developmental nature of the condition with late emerging
motor signs makes early identification of cerebral palsy a diagositc challenge. There is obviously no early pathognomonic sign, x-ray, or laboratory

test which in itself is confirmatory. Evidence to substantiate a diagnosis must be gathered in an orderly and consistent sequential way with full knowledge of the total maturation process rather than fixation on a focal neurological or physical deficit. This is the developmental approach to diagnosis.

One must start with concern about risk and an index of suspicion. The beginning point is often the pediatrician, family practitioner, or other health professional who is consulted by a concerned parent whose child is not making normal progress in motor milestones or speech. Too often the matter may not be given serious consideration if definite local motor abnormality is not found. The parent may be reassured and told to return if no progress is forthcoming, in the hope that delayed development will ultimately speed up and resume a normal pattern. A similar situation may occur as well in a highly sophisticated neonatal intensive care unit from which an infant is discharged following treatment for respiratory distress syndrome. Difficulty in feeding and ordinary infant management when brought to the attention of medical staff on follow-up clinic visits may be attributed to immaturity, poor organization at home, or emotional upset within the family environment.

In fact, each of these situations may represent a child with significant developmental delays due to a fixed motor lesion which ultimately will appear as one of the major motor forms of cerebral palsy. Parental concern may well be appropriate while the professional response is dilatory or nonexistent.

Professional awareness is the starting point in early diagnosis and must be based upon a sensitivity to possible neurological deficit in any child with developmental delay or infant behavior problems. The basis of parental concern must be probed further, rather than merely looking for discrete structural or neurological abnormality. Knowledge of the developmental process needs to be incorporated into the professional's function and used appropriately as any other diagnostic tool. Only in this way will it be possible to develop a realistic and appropriate sense of whether a child is in fact at risk of cerebral palsy or other developmental disability. The index of suspicion should then generate initiation of a full process of developmental evaluation— and not physical examination alone. This should be recorded on a form such as that illustrated in Appendix B.

A systematic and uniform multifactor developmental evaluation approach to early diagnosis is essential to identify the specific diagnosis (if possible) in children who clearly have a nonprogressive developmental disability. The suggested procedure is referred to as the Infant Developmental Evaluation Profile (Table 1). Its features are explored in detail in the following sections.

Table 1   Infant Developmental Evaluation Profile

    I. Developmental history
       Family/genetic
       Pregnancy/labor/delivery
       Perinatal and neonatal
       Behavioral soft signs
       Developmental milestones
   II. Developmental physical examination
  III. Developmental neurological examination
       Tone
       Reflex behavior
          Primitive
          Postural
       Focal signs
       Neurologic soft signs

Developmental History

The chief complaint or concern of the parent presents the intial focus.
Often, this is diffuse and sometimes disorganized, with confusion about
the actual problem. "Advice" from friends and relatives, and poorly understood information gleaned from the media may greatly color the real
issues. The time-consuming procedure of directing and putting into order these concerns may discourage even the most patient examiner.
Skillful and well-directed interviewing, however, will channel unrelated
or even diffuse information into a pattern which is digestable and able
to be integrated into the history to follow. The examiner shold elicit
not only the area of most concern but the age and circumstances at
which the problem was first noted. This will be of help in guiding discussion about the needs of the family.

An accurate and complete history is the first step in the process of developmental evaluation. Adequate records must be obtained where possible.
However, birth and hospital records may not be sufficiently detailed or accurate, particularly if obstetrical or neonatal events have been complex or
traumatic. On the other hand, reliability and possible bias of the parent or
guardian should be weighed in assessing the information given. It is important to obtain information using a well-organized, logical sequence of questions, so that gaps or omissions will be minimal. Factors which may be of
significance are discussed below.

Family and Genetic History

Parental and sibling health should be reviewed, particularly as it relates to the prepregnancy period. Endocrine and metabolic disorders such as thyroid, pituitary abnormality, or diabetes may be relevant. History of seizures and other central nervous system (CNS) problems should be detailed. These would include any evidence of previous mental retardation, learning disorders, attention deficits, cerebral palsy, seizures, emotional disorders, congenital malformations, or multiple handicapping conditions among any family members. Evidence for any genetic disease should be elicited, particularly possible patterns of genetic developmental transmission. These may include such conditions as Down's syndrome, Sturge-Weber syndrome and related disorders, genetic forms of cerebral palsy, and evidence for familial organic learning disorders or varieties of mental retardation.

Pregnancy

Quality of the pregnancy is important and relates to feelings of well-being or anxiety, presence of bleeding, health problems, and fetal movements. Each of these may give an indication of pertinent abnormality. Persistent bleeding may indicate intrauterine developmental abnormality, especially if it occurred early. Infection, toxemia, and use of medication such as diuretics, anticonvulsants, and various types of antibiotics may be of importance. Late onset or diminished fetal movement may indicate a poorly developing fetus. History of possible trauma or stress should be carefully evaluated.

Length of gestation and the presence of prematurity may be crucial. It is often difficult to obtain an accurate history of pregnancy length due to conflicting dates and various obstetrical calculation methods. Every effort should be made to document possible premature gestation to assess better the relation to birth weight and the extent of developmental risk.

Labor and Delivery

Details of labor should include extent of labor before delivery and rate of progression. Evidence for dystocia or prolonged labor should be considered as well as precipitate or rapid labor. Either may be of considerable significance. A prolonged period between membrane rupture and delivery could be a basis for fetal infection. Obstetrical features of the delivery must include use of anesthesia, mechanical events such as version, abnormal presentations, use of instrumentation, and rationale for caesarean section if performed. The place of delivery may be relevant, especially if at home en route to the hospital, or under unusual circumstances.

Perinatal and Neonatal Events

Assessment of condition of the child at birth requires information about birth weight, presence of a nuchal cord, respiratory status, the need for prolonged oxygen treatment, continuous apnea, cyanosis, or resuscitative procedures. History is needed of possible sepsis, meningitis, neonatal seizures, and the presence of any type of congenital malformation. Jaundice shortly after birth due to possible blood group incompatibility should be distinguished from subsequent hyperbilirubinemia in the neonatal period possibly related to breast feeding, galactosemia, infection such as hepatitis, or structural abnormality of the liver. Reports of an abnormally small or large head circumference should be given appropriate consideration, for microcephaly or hydrocephaly.

History of progress up to the first month should be selectively examined for an overview of the entire neonatal period. Particular attention is needed to review activity and behavior of the infant, looking for evidence of marked irritability, hyperactivity, limited environmental contact, or interaction with the environment. Feeding activity may be crucial especially if the child sucks or swallows poorly and is thought to have "colic." This may be one of the earliest signs of central nervous system malfunction and represents one of a number of problems in infant organization and adaptation referred to as "behavioral soft signs" and discussed in detail later in this chapter.

Developmental Milestones

The major developmental milestones present an orderly sequence through which the child is expected to progress normally. An arrest or delay at a given stage is usually the basis for initial parental referral. Not uncommonly, this is the reference point from which the examiner must go back and bring into focus a chief complaint as a first step in the developmental evaluation process.

A list of milestones with variation is given in Table 2. It is useful to elicit this information in the following order, specifically inquiring about when each of the modalities was achieved: (a) smiling; (b) head control in prone position, (c) grasping, (d) transferring, (e) sitting; (f) crawling including quality of motion, (g) independent walking with quality of movement and evidence of any deficits.

Oral development should be carefully reviewed including any difficulties in sucking, chewing, tongue thrusting, and drooling, problems in both eruption, enamelization, or jaw structure, and dental development. Onset of speech should be noted, including intelligibility and quality of sounds, with a

Table 2   Normal Development Compared with Average Development of 100 Cerebral Palsy Children

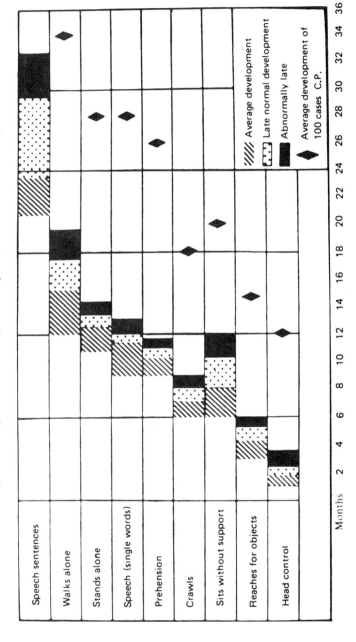

Source: Courtesy of Crippled Children and Adults of Rhode Island, Inc., Providence, Rhode Island

description of progression to phrases and sentences. Verbal behavior is most important, bearing in mind verbosity, repetitive speech, and early evidence of echolalia. Information should also be obtained about hearing acuity and discrimination, visual development, and the onset of and response to environmental stimuli.

The developmental milestones present the major clinical parameter of progressive central nervous system growth and integration. Delay or arrest beyond the normally acceptable range may provide the most significant confirmatory evidence of developmental disability, particularly when considered in conjunction with abnormality in developmental history, including family background, pregnancy, labor, or delivery. No one factor alone will necessarily be definitive, but all taken together can form a framework to establish the diagnosis.

Table 2 also illustrates the significance of developmental milestones contrasting a normal with a population of cerebral palsy patients. Note the wide range of normal appearance in each modality and a very marked delay among the cerebral palsy group.

Other Developmental Features

Social and emotional variables give an insight into personality integration. Attention should be given to temper tantrums, breath-holding, hyperactivity, limited attention span, and ability to separate from family and adjust in new situations. Play interests are important and should be appropriate for age. These will closely correlate with any obvious physical deficits or limitations. Reaction to and participation in group activities such as preschool or nursery classes gives an insight into demands for attention, supervision, and ability to react both physically and socially. Independence in self-care activities should be assessed. These include feeding, undressing and dressing, and toileting. Problems with the latter may have both neurological and emotional aspects which should be carefully weighed. Finally, in the older child, nursery and preschool adjustment and function will provide an early indication of behavioral problems, learning disabilities, or fine motor function, and should be noted.

Review of Systems

Obviously, particular consideration should be given to general medical or health problems, either associated with or related to possible neurological deficit. Examples would include headaches, double vision, unexplained vomiting, lethargy, personality change, or loss of previously achieved function. Any of these could be related to hydrocephalus, an intracranial vascular lesion or neoplasm. Details of any seizure activity should include whether or not they were associated with fever, frequency, duration, and character of the movements. The history must indicate details of previous neurological evaluation with description of electroencephalogram, CAT scan, and other findings, drugs utilized, and results.

Past Medical History

Apart from seizure history, information should include data from any previous neurological, psychological, and developmental evaluations for which appropriate medical records should be obtained. Documentation of medications in use should include rationale and effect. Previous treatment including occupational, physical, and speech therapies should be noted, with details of associated changes and the child's response. Similar data is needed about bracing procedures or assistive devices used and types of surgery performed.

At the conclusion of the developmental history, the examiner should indicate an impression of parental interest, attitude, and ability to deal with the child. During the course of the interview it is generally possible to arrive at some awareness of these interpersonal factors which can later provide a basis for needed supportive services.

The Developmental Physical Examination

The setting of the examination is important and should provide a relaxed, unhurried atmosphere for parent and child. Obtained measurements of height, weight, and head circumference should be plotted on appropriate standards and analyzed.

Observation of the child gives the first indication of environmental response, social interaction, and relation to parent. Much of this can be done while the developmental history is obtained. Evidence should be noted for possible visual or hearing deficits, and the quality of verbal response or speech. Level and appropriateness of activity and behavior can also be gauged.

Structural abnormalities must be detailed in an orderly manner through examination of skin, head and neck, trunk, abdomen, back, spine, and extremities. Obvious malformations could immediately identify such conditions as Down's syndrome, Sturge-Weber syndrome, neurofibromatosis, tuberous sclerosis, hydrocephalus, meningomyelocele, encephalocele, hemiplegia, and brachial plexus paralysis [21]. Many other minor structural deviations may also be apparent early. Some may be part of a syndrome complex such as abnormal facial features in fetal alcohol syndrome. Others more frequently will not form part of a specific classification but their presence may suggest associated central nervous system malformation.

Examination of the head and neck should include a check for size and shape of fontanelles, cleft palate or lip, structural problems of tongue, mouth, and jaw, and abnormal set or configuration of the ears. This is not unusual in children with multiple anomalies and severe developmental deficit.

Examination of the eyes is not as difficult in small children as might be anticipated if the parent assists. The procedure may be most rewarding. Readily obtainable peripheral eye findings may include strabismus, hypertelorism, epicanthus, cataracts, congenital glaucoma, heterochromia, corneal ring (Wilson's disease), depigmented iris of albinism, blue sclerae of osteogenesis imperfecta, scleral pigmentary deposits with ochronosis, or a cloudy cornea noted in mucopolysaccharidosis.

The fundi must be carefully examined for evidence of retinal inflammation as in rubella, toxoplasmosis, or cytomegalovirus infections. Retinal degeneration may indicate a nonspecific degenerative condition, or retinitis pigmentosa, while macular degeneration is specific for Tay-Sachs disease, Nieman-Pick disease, and Gaucher's disease. Also to be noted are retinal changes indicative of intracranial pressure due to hydrocephalus or tumor, and evidence of possible vascular lesions or malformation.

Neck examination should consider signs of webbing and shortening associated with Klippel-Feil syndrome, platybasia and basilar impression, or possible Turner's syndrome. Congenital torticollis is seen in conjunction with other anomalies, and enlarged thyroid is of major concern. Also, a check should be made for bruits both in the neck and head, for vascular malformations.

Chest evaluation should consider anomalies of the bony thorax such as pectus excavatum and carinium, absent ribs, or aplasia of the pectoralis muscles. Lungs and heart should be assessed for normal functioning.

Abdominal fullness or asymmetry may suggest hydronephrosis associated with renal anomalies, Wilms' tumor, or neuroblastoma. Enlarged liver or spleen would give rise to many diagnostic considerations relating to developmental abnormality including biliary atresia, galactosemia, or Wilson's disease; hemoglobinopathy such as in sickle cell anemia or thalassemia, or congenital red cell abnormality in spherocytosis. Hernia is a common finding, often seen in connection with other malformations.

Genitalia should be noted for ambiguity, abnormality in size or shape, testicular descent, presence of hypo- or epispadius. Evidence of precocious puberty may indicate an intracranial lesion or endocrine malfunction.

Extremities should be examined for poly- or syndactyly, abnormal palmar creases seen in Down syndrome, shortening or asymmetry present in hemiplegia or hemihypertrophy. The hips must be carefully assessed for possible dislocation.

Observation of the back should check for lumbosacral hemangioma, anomalous hair, dermal sinus, or raised lesion consistent with meningomyelocele. Spinal deviation including fixed scoliosis, kyphosis, or excessive lordosis needs further review.

Developmental Neurological Examination

The child's activity in relating to the environment is the point of departure. This may be assessed during the physical examination, special emphasis being given to awareness, interest in the environment and examiner, irritability, attention span, and evidence for hyperactivity. Observation of gross motor function and posture can also be done simultaneously and should include head, neck, and trunk control, sitting, crawling, standing, walking, and hand use. Attention to patterns of movement may indicate the presence of asymmetry consistent with hemiplegia, or excessive movement in dystonia. Character of the cry, voice, and quality of speech are also readily apparent.

Tone should be assessed early in the examination when the child is most relaxed. A useful method is to pull the arms forward to sitting and standing positions of the supine child and observe ability to maintain head and neck upright and stabilize the trunk. Obvious hypotonicity will be apparent. On the other hand, maintenance of the hyperextended trunk and rigid standing with support in the very young infant may be the earliest indication of pathological hypertonus. Distinction should be made between tone of extremities and trunk and any disparity noted. A pattern of hypertonic extremities with hypotonicity of the trunk may be an indication of underlying dystonia which will emerge as athetosis. The ability of a newborn to dorsiflex the foot completely onto the shin is considered normal and any restriction may suggest excessive abnormal tone [Ref. 22 and (Fig. 1)]. Degree of head lag has been quantitated as a standardized reference for comparison with the norm [23].

The floppy child seems to have relatively little control or influence of one joint upon another. Such a finding raises the possibility of a wide differential diagnosis including mental retardation, cerebral palsy, and varieties of myopathies. Generally, children who are extremly hypertonic early and who show an ultimate cerebral palsy diagnosis may eventually have the athetoid form, while those with initial hypotonia may later become spastic [24].

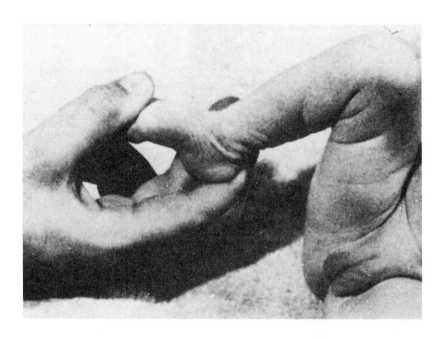

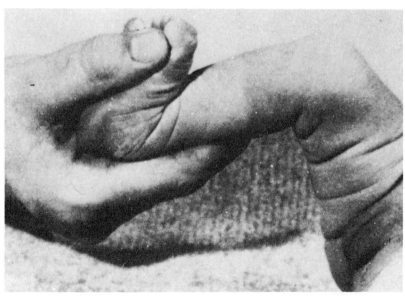

Figure 1   A normal newborn can dorsiflex the foot right onto the shin (from Ref. 4. © 1966, the Williams & Wilkins Co., Baltimore).

Reflex behavior provides a major assessment of brain stem function and CNS developmental integration. It may provide the earliest indication of fixed motor deficit consistent with cerebral palsy long before any discrete motor signs are present. Two major categories function dynamically as the nervous system develops toward maturation of higher centers. The first is a group of *primitive reflexes* present at birth and without which the infant would not be viable. These normally disappear by four to six months with maturation as the *postural reflexes* become manifest and remain life long. The latter are closely associated with and underlie rolling, sitting, crawling, and walking.

The major primitive reflexes which have been described include startle reflex, Moro reflex, rooting, sucking, truncal incurvation, asymmetrical tonic neck reflex, crossed extension, tonic labyrinthine reflex, and others. Since a large number of primitive reflexes are present, there is controversy concerning which have the greatest clinical meaning and predictive significance. Dagarssies places relatively little importance upon truncal incurvation but considers crossed extension to be critical in maturation [12]. Capute et al., on the other hand, include truncal incurvation among the major predictive reflexes being intensely evaluated in an extensive long-range study [25].

Our own clinical experience has led us to give major consideration to the following primitive reflexes in the diagnositc evaluation: startle, Moro, palmar grasp, rooting, sucking, and asymmetric tonic neck (Fig. 2a-e). Weak expression such as poor rooting, sucking, or limited Moro response, would be consistent with abnormality, particularly if there is associated asymmetry. Any persistence beyond 4 to 6 months would provide a strong index of suspicion for significant fixed motor brain deficit—particularly in association with an abnormal developmental history. A strong asymmetric tonic neck reflex (ATNR) is always abnormal especially if the child cries in this position. A strong and persistant ATNR is frequently later associated with athetoid cerebral palsy [26].

A number of postural reflexes are also identified whose diagnostic significance is yet to be fully established. Among those found to be clinically relevant are neck righting, parachute or protective extension, and the Landau reflex. An overview of developmental reflex behavior is shown in Table 3 including the pattern of disappearance of the primitive reflexes and appearance of postural reflexes. Each of these should be tested during the diagnostic evaluation and considered in relation to timing, strength of expression, and symmetry. Differential diagnostic features of abnormal reflex behavior will be discussed in detail later in the chapter. Delayed disappearance of primitives and appearance of posturals is consistent with cerebral palsy;

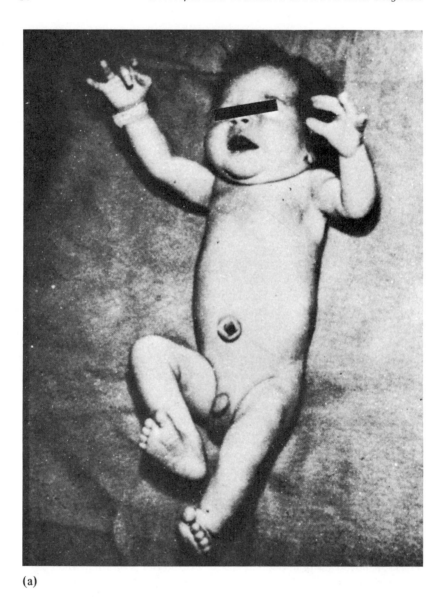

(a)

Figure 2 Primitive reflexes that persist beyond 4-6 months which may indicate fixed motor brain deficiency: (a) Moro reflex; (b) Palmar grasp reflex (a and b from Ref. 4, © 1966, The Williams & Wilkins Co., Baltimore).

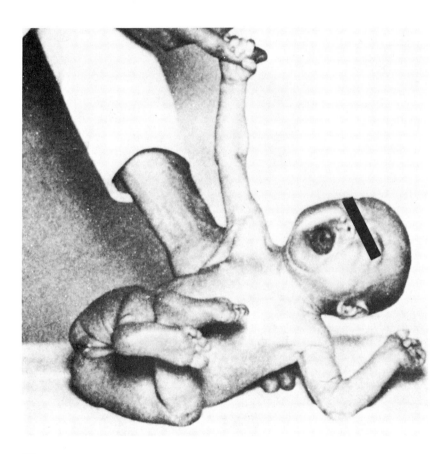

(b)

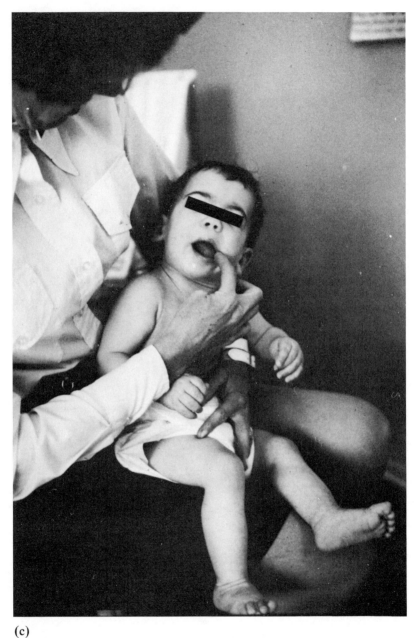

(c)

Figure 2 (continued) Primitive reflexes that persist beyond 4-6 months which may indicated fixed motor brain deficiency: (c) rooting reflex; (d) suckling reflex.

40

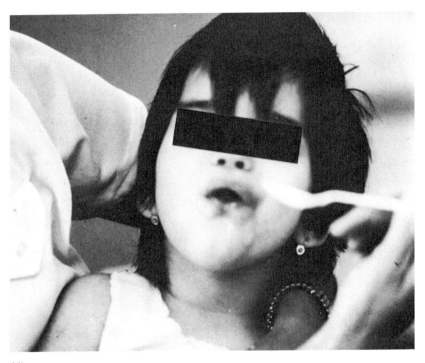

(d)

Figure 2 (continued).

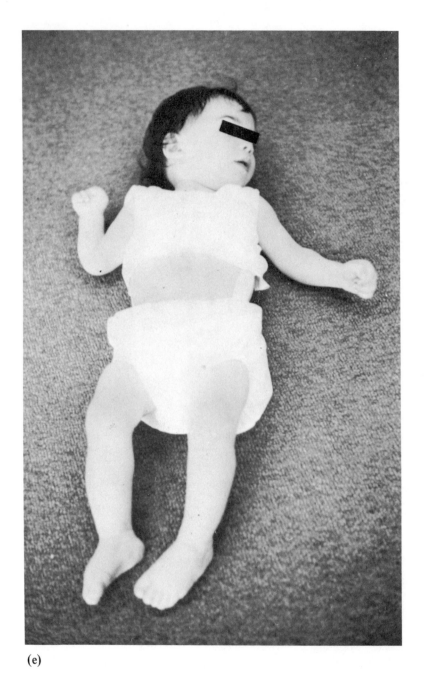

(e)

Figure 2 (continued) Primitive reflexes that persist beyond 4–6 months which may indicate fixed motor brain deficiency: (e) Abnormally delayed ATNR.

normal primitive disappearance and delayed posturals is characteristic of
mental retardation [27]. The entire primitive and postural mechanism is
discussed in further detail in Chapters 4 and 5. Particular attention is given
to association with tone, reciprocal innervation, and patterns of posture and
movement.

Sensory modalities should include response to touch and pain. Where indicated, specific responses at various dermatome levels should be obtained as
in possible lower motor lesions.

Cranial nerve evaluation may be difficult in small children. From a developmental point of view an accurate observation of III, IV, and VI can be obtained for evidence of strabismus; V for mandibular function, and with VII
for corneal reflex and facial asymmetry, IX and XI for swallowing and gag
reflex, XII function may be possible to estimate especially if there is tongue
deviation.

Cerebellar dysfunction may be equally difficult to recognize in the infant
and very small child. Exaggerated opticokinetic nystagmus should be elicited
using response to horizontal movements. Ataxia may be indicated through
observation of balance of head, neck, and trunk, and demonstration of hand
use with small objects.

Dystonia is often subtle and difficult to identify. Disparity of tone between trunk and extremities may be the first suggestive sign, particularly if
there is significant hypotonicity of the trunk. This may quickly alternate to
truncal hypertonicity. Stiffness and hyperextension of the entire body, but
particularly of the face, head, and upper limbs, may dramatically change.
Apparent limitation in range of motion in the extremities may give way to
full movement and no restriction if the child can be relaxed. In the slightly
older patient, facial movements and grimacing may be observed together with
movements of the upper limbs and an overpronated position of arms and
hands. Variable tone remains a cardinal feature which may involve trunk and
extremities. Depending upon the state of the child, these features may vary
from time to time, especially in early developmental stages. Actual dys-
tonic movement characteristic of athetosis is likely to appear very late, whereas the early stiffness judged too rapidly before the child is relaxed is often
misdiagnosed as spasticity. Variability in findings related to athetosis has also
played a part in the past confusion of cerebral palsy classification (see Chap.
1) particularly relating to "types" of athetosis, and the relation to the tremor,
atonia, rigidity, and even ataxia. The clinical distinction between these can
be most difficult in a very small child.

Upper motor neuron signs relating to the motor area and pyramidal tracts
can generally be elicited without difficulty, particularly if there is asym-

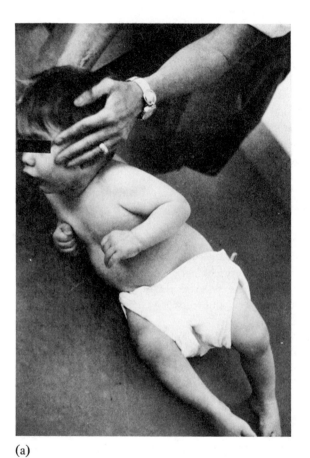

(a)

Figure 3   Postural reflexes of diagnostic and prognostic significance: (a) neck righting reflex; and (b) protective extension (parachute reflex). (From R. S. Paine, Neurological examination of infants and children. *Pediatr. Clin. North Am.* 7:471, 1960).

metry. Markedly exaggerated deep tendon reflexes can be judged accurately indicating evidence for spasticity. Babinski sign may be variable and often cannot be definitely evaluated. Its significance even in newborns is also questioned since it may not be found at all [28]. Frequently, clonus can

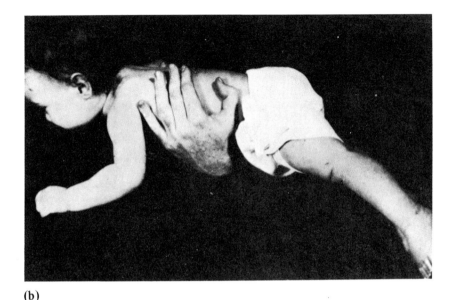

(b)

best be demonstrated by placing the child in the prone position and gently dorsiflexing the great toe or anterior part of the foot. This maneuver tends to displace voluntary motor activity away from the feet so that the reflex is not dampened.

Soft signs refer to a group of functional neurological findings which are general and not focal, often subtle, and may relate to faulty integration in abnormal development [29]. They give clues to underlying poor organization and possible central nervous system deficit. Early on they are manifest as "behavioral" soft signs and later may be identified as discrete neurological abnormalities in fine motor and integrative functioning. One of the earliest may affect sucking, swallowing, and feeding and has already been mentioned in connection with neonatal "colic." Persistent irritability, demanding behavior, continuous gross movement and activity, markedly limited attention span, delayed speech with poor or repetitive expression, withdrawn and isolated behavior, irregular sleep habits, may all suggest underlying deficit in the

Table 2   Infant Reflexes and Age (Month) Normally Demonstrated

Months	1	2	3	4	6	9	12	15	18	24
Primitive										
Moro	+	+	±	±	0	0	0	0	0	0
Palmar	+	+	±	±	0	0	0	0	0	0
ATNR	+	+	±	±	0	0	0	0	0	0
Rooting/suck	+	+	+	±	±	0	0	0	0	0
Postural										
Neck right	0	0	0	±	±	+	+	+	+	+
Parachute	0	0	0	0	±	+	+	+	+	+
Landau	0	0	0	0	0	0	+	+	+	±

infant. For the older child, a systematic approach to observing other of these features is indicated during examintion if the subject is capable of some cooperation. This would include visual tracking without moving the head, blowing out the cheeks, lateralizing the tongue, demonstrating fine finger movements, rapid succession movements, and at a later stage identifying self and other person laterality.

The soft signs add another dimension to the diagnostic capability by either confirming impressions from other positive motor findings or suggesting areas other than gross motor as sources of developmental deficit. These might include mental retardation, attention deficit disorder, autism, or emotional disorder. More specifically, directed diagnostic assessments could then be undertaken.

Screening estimates of psychological functioning are an important aspect of the initial developmental evaluation. Various professionals other than the psychologist can undertake or supplement this function. The Denver Developmental Screening Test is easily administered in a short time by the physician or other professional, and provides a visually descriptive index of functioning in fine and gross motor, language, and social skills [30]. It has the added advantage of being easily updated and provides a visual impression of change.

For the older child who is capable of using paper and pencil, a figure copy test is useful to give gross estimates of developmental levels, visual-perceptual-motor deficits, ability to follow directions, and degree of attention span. A modified figure copy test with levels of function is given in Appendix C with associated developmental levels.

The Goodenough test, in which the child of three or older is directed to draw a person may also be administered [31]. This provides an indication of developmental level and may also give some insight into the degree of personality integration and concentration ability of the child. Like the figure copy test, it has the advantage of being easily administered during the developmental examination by the physician or other health personnel.

The Scope of Laboratory Evaluation

The extent to which laboratory procedures are needed to aid in diagnosis will depend upon findings of the physical and neurological examinations in relation to the developmental history. In the child with a history of prematurity and neonatal anoxia who is markedly delayed in milestones and has signs of generalized spasticity, relatively few laboratory data are needed to support a diagnosis of cerebral palsy. However, a patient who has a normal birth history and marked progressive developmental delay with a paucity of findings, would require hospitalization for an extensive work-up. Considerable variation generally exists in the average case. A major benefit of an organized, sequential system of developmental evaluation is that it provides a focus and direction in the usual office or clinic setting which will help to determine the extent to which more detailed work-up will be indicated. The child with a developmental delay must not be the subject of a shot-gun approach using laboratory findings to determine whether a lesion exists. Rather, the dynamic and changing nature of the central nervous system, especially one in which there is some deficit, has to be viewed in its entirety.

Screening tests which may be useful initially include complete blood count and urinalysis, serum lead levels, T4/TSH for thyroid function, urinary amino acid study, Torch titer, and skull x-rays for evidence of intracranial calcification. Even these procedures should be limited unless clinically indicated.

The electroencephalogram is much abused and frequently misused. It is clearly indicated and should be mandatory where there is a seizure history and may be of considerable assistance in management. Where there is behavior disorder or hyperactivity, it generally has little to add. As a routine procedure it has no place and should be discouraged. Unfortunately, many teachers and others who deal professionally with children have come to regard it as a major developmental diagnostic tool. They often need guidance and direction to discourage this approach. A similar situation seems to be emerging with computerized axial tomography (CAT scan) and magnetic resonance imaging (MRI). These highly effective procedures may be vital in the work-up of a child with significant developmental delays. However, their use must be first based upon considerations derived from an orderly and systematic approach.

FORMULATING THE DIAGNOSIS

Cerebral Palsy

As pointed out earlier, the very young child with a fixed motor lesion will not show focal signs of spasticity, athetosis, ataxia, or mixed patterns. Rather, there will initially be abnormalities of tone, persistence of primitive reflex activity with delay in disappearance, and late, often incomplete, emergence of postural reflexes. Developmental history is crucial in diagnosis. Paucity of laboratory findings is to be expected. Where the developmental history is strongly positive and signs of abnormal tone and reflex behavior are present a probable diagnosis of cerebral palsy is appropriate. Utilizing this sequential developmental evaluation procedure will allow a definite diagnosis within the first few months of life and a presumptive one even earlier.

Again, it must be emphasized that in the very young child and infant the traditional motor forms of cerebral palsy are generally not present. These gradually emerge during the first year and beyond as the abnormal nervous system matures. The condition in very young children may appear merely as a nonspecific form of developmental delay. However, using the above features of developmental evaluation it is indeed possible to formulate at least a probable diagnosis of cerebral palsy long before the definitive motor manifestations are apparent.

In the older child, generally beyond one year, a diagnosis of cerebral palsy can often be made indicating a specific motor type. This may change as the child grows and the definitive motor defect becomes more apparent. Definitive motor signs may also disappear early in very mild cases. As the child grows, it is possible to formulate specifics of extent and degree of involvement, namely, cerebral palsy, spastic quadriplegia, mild upper involvement, moderate lower involvement. Where possible, it is useful to include these features in the diagnosis so that some prognostic outlook is available.

Developmental Delay

It is not always practical nor desirable to place a diagnostic label on a child. When dealing with the very young nervous system, it is often not possible to have complete assurance that developmental history and physical and neurological evaluations are clearly compatible with cerebral palsy, or other specific recognizable entity. However, evidence for definite and significant developmental delay may be present and the judgment or maturity of the examiner will then determine the subsequent course. It is at this point that parents not infrequently are told by the physician that the child will "grow out of it." The later outcome may indeed confirm the initial parental concern. More predictable identification is achievable if the systematic process of developmental evaluation is followed regularly by the professional.

Nevertheless, an examiner is sometimes hesitant to inform parents of possible deficit because of uncertainty about the diagnosis, not being aware of what treatment is available, or not convinced of its effectiveness. The rapid rise of early intervention programs and increasing evidence of significant effect for child and family (see Chap. 9) are compelling reasons to put this latter factor to rest.

Practitioners may be concerned about unduly alarming parents, believing that a gradual approach over time will be less distressing. Perhaps in time the parents will see for themselves that the child is abnormal and seek help. To be guided by either of these possibilities places the family in severe emotional jeopardy. They are already concerned or would not have come for the evaluation. Without guidance and direction they are likely to seek other opinions and will face further uncertainty and confusion from "shopping around" and obtaining a variety of judgments. Too often, this leads to severe emotional conflict and major adjustment problems within a family.

When some doubt exists about an exact diagnosis or confirmation of cerebral palsy cannot be made with certainty it is best to inform parents that the child shows definite developmental delay without using a specific label. This sets the stage for future action. It may confirm what the parents know already and return balance and stability to the family. A plan of action is decided upon and should include referral for some form of early intervention program. It also keeps open possibilities for future development and demands that the child be seen at regular periodic intervals to monitor change. Continuity of follow-up by the same professional group is essential if at all practical to assess needs and progress fully. Only in this way will it be possible to provide adequate communication with and support for parents and plan appropriately for the future. The need for continuous reevaluation does not cease even when a specific diagnosis of a cerebral palsy type can be made. Cerebral palsy is always a presumptive diagnosis since confirmatory evidence is indirect and is based upon behavior and development at a given time. One must always be on guard for any changes which may be consistent with progressive disease, however subtle or slow in nature. This is particularly true of cerebellar or mixed cerebral palsy lesions.

Some classification other than static encephalopathy is helpful to characterize the dynamic and changing developmental deficit which is identified early before a specific diagnosis is possible. The categories in Table 4 are suggested for use with the young child. Such a classification could provide uniformity in description and greatly improve interprofessional communication.

Categories 2 and 3 would require referral for an intervention program and continuous reevaluation. Many cases would subsequently be placed in a cerebral palsy or other specific diagnostic category.

The recognition of significant developmental deficit in the young child will lead to planning an appropriate program (see Chap. 3). This should be twofold. The first consideration is management: to develop specific techniques and procedures in caring for the child. These are necessary because deficits may severely limit and alter the usual child care regime. Second, simultaneous treatment or therapy is instituted to guide and stimulate a more normal pattern of neurological development and growth. Both manage-

Table 4 Early Developmental Deficit Classification

1. Normal child—mild developmental immaturity
2. Developmental delay
   a. Motor
   b. Oral/Speech
   c. Cognitive
   d. Behavior
3. Developmental abnormality—nonspecific
   a. Motor
   b. Oral/Speech
   c. Cognitive
   d. Behavior (severity)
      1. Mild
      2. Moderate
      3. Profound

ment and treatment constitute the early intervention program which can be offered for the infant with a nonspecific developmental deficit diagnosis as well as the young child with specifically identified cerebral palsy. The process should be continuous and flexible enough to deal with the neurological lesion as it becomes increasingly apparent and discrete.

DIFFERENTIAL DIAGNOSTIC CONSIDERATIONS

Nonprogressive Developmental Deficits

Congenital Cerebral Palsy

The following features of congenital cerebral palsy in infancy can be readily identified utilizing the Infant Developmental Evaluation Profile (Table 1):

History: There is generally some *positive* history of abnormality in pregnancy, labor, or delivery, such as prematurity, respiratory, or other significant difficulty in the neonatal period. Behavioral *soft signs*, particularly in the neonatal period, are frequently found. They include colicky behavior with significant irritability, frequent problems in feeding, and failure to develop regular sleep patterns. The combination of a significant pregnancy or birth history with colic-like behavior or sleep disturbance is often the most powerful predictor that the developmental delay is indeed cerebral palsy.

Developmental Milestones: It is important to recognize the well-established sequential nature of motor developmental milestones as well as the broad range of their appearance and disappearance (Table 2). The cerebral palsied child will be significantly delayed in reaching milestones. Generally speaking, the child comes to the attention of the physician when there has been some delay in reaching milestones. The degree of delay must be assessed and considered in relation to abnormalities in the history and the possible presence of soft signs in order to heighten the index of suspicion.

Physical examination in the infant with cerebral palsy generally will not yield specific findings. The exception is the situation in which there is motor asymmetry. Frequently the infant has had delay both in growth and development and may show a failure to thrive syndrome.

Neurological Examination: Emphasis should be on awareness, relatedness, and responsiveness of the child. Adequacy of vision and hearing are of particular importance and should be assessed clinically. Of major concern are *abnormalities of tone*. Generally, infants with cerebral palsy have tone disturbances, either of hypotonia with floppiness and poor control of head, neck, and trunk, or a stiffness and rigidity. Sometimes the latter is noted early by the parent and considered an expression of advanced development because the child is early able to be brought to a standing position. In fact, stiffness and hypertonia may be one of the earliest indicators of significant neuromotor abnormalities.

Reflex behavior represents a powerful predictive feature in diagnosing the cerebral palsy infant (Table 3) [32]. Most often, primitive reflexes will be *delayed in disappearance* in cerebral palsy [27]. There may also be abnormalities in their expression. For example, a very strong or obligatory asymmetric tonic neck reflex is almost pathognomonic in cerebral palsy, particularly athetosis. Depending upon the degree of severity, there may be variable expressions of several of the primitive reflexes initially in the infant with cerebral palsy, that is, an inadequate or incomplete Moro, poor rooting, or sucking.

Equally important is the *delay in appearance* or incomplete expression of the postural reflexes [33]. This combination of delay in disappearance of the primitive reflexes with variable expression and delay in the appearance of postural reflexes is a powerful predictor of cerebral palsy. This is especially true when viewed in relation to the totality of abnormal findings of the Development Evaluation Profile including abnormalities in tone, delays in achieving milestones, the presence of soft signs, and an abnormal history.

It is essential to bear in mind that the specific motor forms of cerebral palsy appear late as the abnormal central nervous system matures. Focal neurological signs other than asymmetry are not generally seen in the infant. Instead one must rely on more indirect indicators and multiple variables, such as the features included in the Infant Developmental Evaluation Profile.

Acquired cerebral palsy will be identified by specific fixed motor type in a child who had previously been normal and after a specific brain insult. Preceding features of tone, primitive or postural reflex behavior, and milestones all would have been appropriate.

In *genetic cerebral palsy*, few data are available concerning the rare cases of genetic cerebral palsy. In contrast with congenital types, tone and primitive reflexes are nearer normal, while there is delay in postural reflexes and specific abnormality in milestones, namely, delayed or absent walking in familial spastic paraplegia. There may be a family history of similar cases [34].

MENTAL RETARDATION/ATTENTION DEFICIT DISORDER

Specific Differential Diagnosis The features of the Infant Developmental Evaluation Profile are summarized in Table 5 and enable comparison of cerebral palsy with characteristics of the infant with mental retardation or

Table 5 Developmental Disabilities: Early Differential Diagnosis Features

	Cerebral Palsy (CP)	Mental retardation (MR)	Attention deficit hyperactivity disorder (ADHD)
I. History	Often positive	Generally negative	Possible family, especially males
A. Soft signs	Colic; irritable; sleep problems	"Easy baby"	Active; demand; colic; sleep problems
B. Milestones	Delayed	Delayed	Advanced motor; Delayed speech
II. Physical exam	Negative Delayed growth	Negative or syndrome	Negative
III. Neurological evaluation			
A. Tone	Increased or decreased	Hypotonia	Normal
B. Reflex behavior			
1. Primitive	Persists	Normal disappearance	Normal disappearance
2. Postural	Delayed appearance	Delayed appearance	Early appearance
C. Focal signs	Appear late	Absent	Absent

attention deficit/hyperactivity disorder. It will be seen that in mental retardation there is generally a negative history. The child is often "too easy"
to deal with and does not have feeding problems or sleep disturbances. Significant delay in milestones is present, and there is generally hypotonia.
Finally, a major differential point is the *normal disappearance* of primitive
reflexes and *significant delay in the appearance* of postural reflexes [35].
For the infant with attention deficit/hyperactivity disorder a positive family
history of hyperactivity or learning disabilities may be noted, especially in
the father, or in siblings. There may be some evidence of colic or sleep problems, but the child is often very active and demanding in behavior. Motor
milestones may be *significantly advanced*. However, there is frequently a
noticeable delay in developing speech patterns. Finally, the reflex behavior
shows both normal disappearance of the primitives and frequently early appearance of the postural reflexes.

ORGANIC BRAIN SYNDROMES/EMOTIONAL DISORDERS

At times, the child with organic brain syndrome is withdrawn and exhibits
autisticlike qualities, having little contact either socially or interpersonally.
Under these circumstances it is often difficult to differentiate levels of development or achievement of milestones. This is equally true of the child
with primary emotional disorder. Here the tested reflex behavior would be
appropriate. Milestones, particularly those involving speech may be delayed.

Progressive CNS Disease

Progressive CNS disease must be given serious consideration when there are
delays in development, the pregnancy and birth history is normal, no abnormalities are found on examination, yet there is marked abnormality or delay
in reflex behavior or milestones. This would be particularly true if earlier
milestones had been normal and subsequent development is abberant.
Hydrocephalus with persistent increased intracranial pressure should be
seriously considered in children with full, open fontanelles and a markedly
enlarged cranial circumference. Neoplasia or vascular malformations must
also be ruled out in this situation.

The progressive lipoidoses would be evident by the cherry red macula in
Tay-Sachs and Niemann-Pick diseases, and hyperpigmented yellow retinal
lesions in Gaucher's disease. Cloudy cornea may be seen in mucopolysac-
charidoses, corneal ring in Wilson's disease, and blue sclerae in osteogenesis
imperfecta. Primitive and postural reflexes have not been well-studied in

these cases but would vary considerably with degree of involvement. All would show delay in appearance of postural reflexes and milestones.

Lesch-Nyhan syndrome occurs in boys in association with high uric acid levels and a specific enzyme defect [36]. Positive family history is frequently noted. Unexplained high fevers are present and severe self-mutilation develops early. Without restraint, amputation of fingers will occur. At 12 to 18 months, typical severe generalized athetosis appears and has been frequently diagnosed as the congenital variety. Unfortunately in this instance the condition is progressive and the prognosis grave.

Other nonspecific progressive disorders of grey or white matter should be considered where the history is normal in association with marked subsequent developmental delay. Pelizaeus-Merzbacher disease and a variety of leukodystrophies will be arrived at by exclusion. Alexander's disease is identified by progressive macrocephaly without increased intracranial pressure.

Neuropathies are rare in young children and generally would not be a differential consideration. An infectious polyneuritis with significant functional residua could be considered when onset is acute and infection can be documented. Anterior horn cell infection as in poliomyelitis is generally identifiable without difficulty. Degeneration of the anterior horn cell as in Werdnig-Hoffmann disease or variants would be extremely rare, but should be considered.

Myopathies

A spectrum of benign intrinsic muscle disease is now recognized which may be seen in association with the "floppy child" and delayed milestones. These include nemaline myopathy, central core disease, and others [37]. The outcome is generally favorable.

Muscular dystrophy might be a serious consideration in boys beyond the toddler stage who show delay in progression or actual regression in gross motor development. Abnormality in previous reflex behavior or tone would not be expected.

Myasthenia gravis [38] with severe hypotonia may be seen transiently in newborns in association with maternal disease or may be present as a primary disease. The life-threatening nature of the condition is likely to lead to prompt and extensive evaluation.

REFERENCES

1. Gesell, A., and Amatruda, C. Developmental Diagnosis, Normal and Abnormal Child Development, Clinical Methods and Pediatric Applications. New York, Hoeber, 1947.

2. Pascal, G., and Jenkins, W. Systemic Observations of Gross Human Behavior. New York, Grune and Stratton, 1961.

3. Bayley, N. Value and limitations of infant testing. *Children* 5:129,1958.

4. Illingworth, R. The Development of the Infant and Young Child—Normal and Abnormal. Baltimore, Williams & Wilkins, 1966.

5. Jackson, J. Evolution and dissolution of the nervous system. In Taylor, J. (Ed.). Selected Writings of John Hughlings Jackson. Vol. 2. New York, Basic Books, 1958.

6. Bobath, K. The Motor Deficit in Patients with Cerebral Palsy. Little Club Clinics in Developmental Medicine. London, Heinemann, 1966.

7. Peyser, A. Cerebral Function in Infancy and Childhood. New York, Consultants Bureau, 1963.

8. Prechtl, H., and Beintema, D. Neurological Examination of the Full Term Infant. Little Club Clinics in Developmental Medicine, London, Heinemann, 1964.

9. Milani-Camparetti, A. Spasticity versus patterned postural and motor behavior of spastics. *Excerpta Med. Int. Congr. Ser.* 107. IV International Congress of Physical Medicine. Paris, 1964.

10. Sherrington, C. The Integrative Action of the Nervous System. New Haven, Yale University Press, 1961.

11. Clarke, E., and O'Malley, C. The Human Brain and Spinal Cord. Berkeley, University of California Press, 1968.

12. Dargassies, S. Neurological Development in the Full Term and Premature Neonate, New York, Excerpta Medica, 1977.

13. Bobath, B., and Bobath, K. Motor Development in Different Types of Cerebral Palsy. London, Heinemann, 1975.

14. Drillien, C. Abnormal neurologic signs in the first year of life in low birth weight infants: Possible prognostic significance. *Dev. Med. Child. Neurol.* 14:575, 1972.

15. Amiel-Tison, C. Neurological evaluation of the maturity of newborn infants. *Arch. Dis. Child.* 43:89, 1968.

16. Dubowitz, L., Dubowitz, V., and Goldberg, C. Clinical assessment of gestational age in the newborn infant. *J. Pediatr.* 77:1, 1970.

17. Bayley, N. Bayley Scales of Mental and Motor Development, as used in the Collaborative Perinatal Research Project of the National Institute of Neurological Diseases and Blindness, Bethesda, MD, 1961.

18. Reed, H. Review of Peabody Developmental Motor Scales and Activity Cards. In Mitchell, J. (Ed.): The Ninth Mental Measurements Yearbook. Lincoln, University of Nebraska Press, 1985, p. 1119.

19. Kaye, L., and Whitfield, M. The eight month movement assessment of infants as a prediction of cerebral palsy in high risk infants (abstr). *Dev. Med. Child. Neurol.* 30(Suppl 57):11, 1988.

20. Morgan, A. Early diagnosis of cerebral palsy using a profile of abnormal motor patterns (abstr). *Dev. Med. Child. Neurol.* 30(Suppl 57):12, 1988.

21. Rosenthal, R., Scherzer, A., and Cooper, W. Unusual etiologies in congenital cerebral palsy. *Rev. Hosp. Spec. Surg.* 1:36, 1971.

22. Dargassies, S. Le nouveau-Ne a terme. Aspect neurologique. *Biol. Neonate* 4:174, 1962.

23. Thomas, A., Chesni, Y., and Dargassies, S. The Neurological Examination of the Infant. Little Club Clinics in Developmental Medicine. London, Heinemann, 1960.

24. Paine, R. The early diagnosis of cerebral palsy. *R. I. Med. J.* 44:522, 1961.

25. Capute, A., Accardo, P., Vining, E., Rubeinstein, J., and Harryman, S. Primitive Reflex Profile. Baltimore, University Park Press, 1978.

26. Paine, R. The evolution of infantile postural reflexes in the presence of chronic brain syndromes. *Dev. Med. Child. Neurol.* 6:345, 1964.

27. Molnar, G. Motor deficit of retarded infants and young children. *Arch. Phys. Med. Rehab.* 55:393, 1974.

28. Hogan, G., and Milligan, J. The plantar reflex of the newborn. *N. Engl. J. Med.* 285:502, 1971.

29. Paine, R., and Oppé, T. Neurological Examination of Infants and Children. Little Club Clinics in Developmental Medicine. London, Heinemann, 1966, p. 187.

30. Frankenberg, W., Goldstein, A., and Camp, B. The revised Denver Developmental Screening Test: its accuracy as screening instrument. *J. Pediatr.* 79:908, 1971.

31. Harris, D. Children's Drawings as Measures of Intellectual Maturity. New York, Harcourt, Brace and World, 1963.

32. Capute, A., and Biehl, R. Functional developmental evaluation: Prerequisite to habilitation. *Pediatr. Clin. North Am.* 20:3, 1973.

33. Bobath, B., and Bobath, K. Motor Development in Different Types of Cerebral Palsy. Little Club Clinics in Developmental Medicine. London, Heinemann, 1975.

34. Silver, J. Familial spastic paraplegia with amyotrophy of the hands. *Ann. Hum. Genet.* 30:69, 1966.

35. Molnar, G., and Gordon, S. Cerebral palsy: predictive value of selected clinical signs for early prognostication of motor function. *Arch. Phys. Med. Rehabil.* 57:153, 1976.

36. Nyhan, W., Oliver, W., and Lesch, M. A familial disorder of uric acid metabolism and central nervous system function. II *J. Pediatr.* 67:257, 1965.

37. Dubowitz, V. The floppy infant: a paractical approach to classification. *Dev. Med. Child. Neurol.* 10:706, 1968.

38. Scherzer, A. L. The Infant with Cerebral Palsy: An Approach to Identification, Management and Treatment. New York, private printing, 1973.

Appendix A   Child Development from 2 Months Through 2 Years[a]

2 months
  Hands predominantly fisted
  Lifts head up for several seconds while prone
  Startles to loud noise
  Follows with eyes and head over 90 degree arc
  Smiles responsively
  Begins to vocalize single vowel sounds

3 months
  Hands occasionally fisted
  Lifts head up above body plane and holds position
  Holds an object briefly when placed in hand
  Turns head toward object, fixes and follows fully in all directions with eyes
  Smiles and vocalizes when talked to
  Watches own hands, stares at faces
  Laughs

4 months
  Holds head steady while in sitting position
  Reaches for an object, grasps it, brings it to mouth
  Turns head in direction of sound
  Smiles spontaneously

5 to 6 months
  Lifts head while supine
  Rolls from prone to supine
  Lifts head and chest up in prone position
  No head lag
  Transfers object from hand to hand
  Babbles
  Sits with support
  Localizes direction of sound

7 to 8 months
  Sits in tripod fashion without support
  Stands briefly with support
  Bangs object on table
  Reaches out for people
  Mouths all objects
  Says da-da, ba-ba

9 to 10 months
  Sits well without support, pulls self to sit
  Stands holding on
  Waves "bye-bye"
  Drinks from cup with assistance

Appendix A (Continued)

11 to 12 months
Walks holding on
Pincer grasp
Two to four words with meaning
Creeps well
Assists in dressing
Understands a few simple commands

13 to 15 months
Walks by self—falls easily
Says several words, uses jargon
Scribbles with crayon
Points to things wanted

18 months
Climbs stairs holding on, climbs up on chair
Throws ball
Builds two to four block tower
Feed self
Takes off clothes
Points to two to three body parts
Many intelligible words

24 months
Runs, walks up and down stairs alone (both feet per step)
Two to three word sentences
Turns single pages of book
Builds tower of four to six blocks
Kicks ball
Uses pronouns "you," "me," "I"

---

[a]Represents the age at which the average child acquires the skill.
Source: S. B. Brown. The neurologic examination during the first 2 years of life. In. K.F. Swaiman and F. S. Wright, The Practice of Pediatric Neurology. St. Louis, The C. V. Mosby Co., 1975. Data from Refs. 1 and 4.

Appendix B   Initial Developmental Evaluation: Developmental History

---

Date Completed   Informant:

1. Reason for referral: Reliability:

     Age Disability Recognized and Symptoms Noted

2. Family and Genetic History:

3. Pregnancy History:

4. Labor and Delivery:

5. Perinatal and Neonatal Events:
     a. Condition at birth
     b. Neonatal history

6. Developmental Milestones:
     a. Head balance and control
     b. Smiling
     c. Grasping
     d. Transferring
     e. Rolling
     f. Sitting
     g. Crawling
     h. Walking
     i. Hand preference
     j. Oral development
          1. Feeding and sucking
          2. Tongue and mouth problems
          3. Speech
          4. Dental development
     k. Hearing
     l. Vision

7. Other Developmental Features:
     a. Social
     b. Emotional
     c. Play interests
     d. Self-care
          1. Feeding
          2. Dressing
          3. Toileting
     e. School

8. Review of Systems:

9. Past Medical History
   a. Previous evaluations
   b. Medication
   c. Therapy
   d. Braces/equipment
   e. Surgery
10. Parental Attitude and Information:

Appendix C   Developmental Ages

Figure Copying

2-1/2 yrs ◯   7 yrs

3-4 yrs   ✕   8 yrs

5 yrs   ▢   9 yrs

6 yrs   △   10 yrs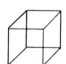

Draw a person test:

3

Planning for the Abnormally Developing Child

CONSEQUENCES OF ABNORMAL NEUROLOGICAL DEVELOPMENT

Discordant Maturation

As we have seen, a nonprogressive deficit of the central nervous system may initially affect the brain stem and influence tone, as well as expression and integrity of primitive or postural reflexes. Motor development and sensory response may equally be impaired. There is considerable variability in the expression of these deficits and uneven developmental growth is frequent. Thus children may respond well to the environment, including visual and auditory stimuli, with a social smile. Yet they might be extremely floppy with an exaggerated primitive reflex pattern. Variable maturational strengths and weaknesses are often a source of confusion in determining whether in fact the child is normal. The apparent discrepancy in response, movement, posture, and reflex behavior may, in fact, be the initial basis for a parent's concern.

The uneven nature of neurological maturation may become even more apparent with physical growth. Varying combinations of deficit may be encountered including floppy or exaggerated tone, immature posture, and abnormal reflexes. Often these characteristics will be present in association with emerging motor problems or asymmetry. Such children are a puzzle to parents. They have some strengths but seem unable to progress in the usual stages. Or perhaps they are seriously limited in all areas but from time to time seem to be making some progress—only to fall back and again be the cause for concern. This is the basis for initial anxiety, often the reason for referral, and generally at the root of tension that may greatly influence inter-family relationships.

The Influence of Abnormal Tone

Excessive floppiness or stiffness of the young child may often be the precipitating cause of concern by the family. A sense of abnormality is frequently conveyed intuitively when the child is somehow recognized to be too flexible and difficult to handle or too rigid to accommodate in the various usual postures.

Hypotonicity is associated with postural limpness and generally severe head lag. Often head, neck, and trunk control are also poor. Difficulties in handling and positioning the child are apparent early. This is initially seen in finding a comfortable, secure posture for feeding, whether by breast or bottle. There is excessive head lag and considerable support is generally necessary for the neck and trunk. This is true in a variety of postures including burping, dressing, bathing, and carrying the child. Floppy infants are immediately at a disadvantage also because they are greatly limited in their physical ability to maintain a secure posture in which to interact with the environment. This could be the start of a long unbroken period of deprivation of contact and stimulation that may add to existing deficits.

Hypertonicity may have similar effects on the child, contact with family, and the environment. It differs in that excessive stiffness is more likely to be viewed as obstinacy by the parent or may be considered causally related to irritability. The possibility of a behavioral factor and emotional stress could be thus introduced early to complicate the picture further. At times, the stiffness enables some degree of "standing" at a very early age and may lead to the erroneous conclusion that the child is excessively mature, and advanced in development.

Often tone will change greatly as the infant develops. As indicated in Chapter 2, it is not infrequent for the hypotonic infant later to become a spastic child or for the initially hypertonic to appear ultimately as an athetoid. Change in tone patterns further confuses the daily problems in management. This is particularly true when the family is sensitive and responsive to adapting to the child.

Finally, there is often variable tone of the trunk and extremities. A hypotonic trunk may be associated with stiff upper extremities as seen in athetosis. Change in position may affect this relationship as well as postural reflexes. The effect is to present much perplexity and many fustrations to those who deal with the child on a daily basis.

Sensory Deficit and Function

The visually impaired infant may have a peripheral deficit such as cataract, congenital glaucoma, or other structural anomaly. The deficit may be central, within the optic tract, or possibly involve the optic cortex. Both types of lesions may also be present. The effect of visual deprivation will be closely related to the complexity of involvement. An intact child with peripheral visual loss alone will obviously not respond to visual stimuli but will be affected by other sensory modalities. In this situation it may be more difficult to identify early that sight is impaired since the child may interact fairly well with the environment.

A central lesion affecting vision is more likely to be associated with other sensory or motor deficits which limit the child's interaction with or appreciation of the surroundings. The limited overall reaction of the child may call attention to developmental abnormality at a very early stage. While the infant may not see in either case, the presence of a peripheral lesion alone does not necessarily block other avenues for contact and learning.

Visual cues expected early in parenteral recognition are missed initially although a smile or verbal response to contact may occur. Within a fairly short time the lack of visual response in feeding confirms the underlying parenteral anxiety. If a central lesion is present, there are likely to be associated abnormalities of tone and reflex behavior as well, further affecting development. At times, it may be quite difficult to determine on observation alone whether visual loss exists, either because the child otherwise interacts well or is totally globally limited. Examination by electroretinography or visually evoked electroencephalography (EEG) may be indicated to ascertain retinal function [1].

Auditory loss is comparable in potentially restricting major environmental contact and the stimulation needed for early development. Extent of overall effect relates to the complexity of deficit—ranging from peripheral (conductive, sensorineuro) to generalized central lesions involving auditory pathways, tone, reflex behavior, and motor abnormalities. Often, hearing loss is not clinically recognized early, particularly if it is peripheral. It may also not be adequately considered in the globally involved child who interacts poorly. A variety of diagnostic procedures may be utilized to delineate the condition, including galvanic skin techniques [2] and the auditory-evoked electroencephalogram [3].

Recent data on hearing loss and emotional and social development confirm a much wider effect than previously had been recognized [4]. This may be beyond the physical and developmental deprivation experienced as a result of limited environmental contact.

The effect, if any, of tactile, proprioceptive, and gustatory loss on the young child has yet to be fully identified. One may speculate that individually or in conjunction with a more complex central lesion, they each could contribute to further deprivation and raise the issue of an appropriate remedial approach. Perceptual deficits and cognitive loss as seen in the learning disabled and mentally retarded, respectively, are limiting factors which restrict the child's options for experience and learning. Those with the greatest deficit have the least resources to utilize other strengths for development. The more mildly involved, however, may be able to use other abilities effectively. Early identification of limitations in these areas is more difficult and the question of how to remediate effectively remains open.

Abnormal Reflex Behavior and Deprivation

In conjunction with other initial neurological deficits abnormalities of primitive and postural reflexes may become major limiting influences on development. The child who roots and sucks poorly will feed poorly. Indeed, a first indication of deficit may be expressed as "colic" and irritability associated with the feeding process related to poor sucking and swallowing, with air trapping and inadequate intake. A strong asymmetric tonic neck reflex will limit reaching out, having contact with textures, shapes, and objects in the environment. Rolling from supine will be delayed or difficult and progression to sitting, crawling, and ambulation will be greatly impeded. Similarly, persistence of the tonic labyrinthine reflex, with associated truncal extension, will delay and limit sitting. Crawling will be restricted by a persisten symmetric tonic neck reflex in which tone of head and upper extremities correspond so that extension of the head will result in extension of the upper limbs and may obstruct movement.

Strongly active and continued primitive reflexes will also influence parents' ability to perform child-care activities. Marked influence is inevitable on positioning, holding, bathing, dressing, and feeding because of abnormal postures and associated easily elicited reflex responses. The implications for management as well as parent-child interaction are obvious and far-reaching. The continued active influence of these and other primitive reflexes serves to "trap" the child in an immature state and intrinsically limit possibilities for self-initiated contact with the environment. Thus, by virtue of the early neurologic defict, the child suffers deprivation of experience and possibly social interaction as well. These problems exist in addition to frequent physical limitations in tone abnormalities and specific motor disorder.

For the slightly older child similar concerns relate to delayed or incomplete appearance of the postural reflexes. Late neck and body righting restricts efforts to roll, sit, and crawl. Limited or incomplete righting reactions affect trunk control, weight bearing, and walking. Here too, delayed expression of reflexes occurs in conjunction with other function-restricting neurological deficits which impair the ability to interact with and actively participate in the environment.

These deficits have an immediate and continuing impact on the child's ability to learn actively from the environment and participate in the process of socialization. Hence, the neurologically impaired child may remain passive, dependent, and out of active contact unless his or her specific developmental needs are recognized and an active stimulation process individually constructed. Implications for both education and socialization of the affected infant relate directly to the inherent restriction from the very beginning of development.

Specific Motor Abnormality: Posture and Movement

The child with a focal motor lesion such as hemiplegia may early show signs of asymmetry. This may be apparent in limited expression of Moro reflex or startle response. Paucity of movement on the affected side will be seen as the child is handled, positioned, and dealt with in all areas of child care. More subtle and generalized motor limitations may be present and will affect movement and limit progression toward the upright posture.

The presence of actual motor signs and restriction will be associated with deficits of tone and reflex behavior. Such a child may well be further limited in physically moving effectively in the environment. Deprivation of contact and the inability to participate actively in the surroundings are serious consequences that may further affect such a child's development.

Oral Development Deficits

Of the many parameters impinging on early maturation, oral development has perhaps the most far-reaching influence. Many dimensions must be considered and full details of evaluation are delineated in Chapter 5. The rapidly emerging literature in this field gives some indication of the extensive areas which must be considered [5-8]. From a functional point of view, the initial concerns relate to limited rooting and sucking reflexes with frequent concomitant inadequate swallowing mechanism. This is not unusual when associated with fixed central nervous system deficit. Inefficient feeding with poor intake and frequent air trapping often results and is accompanied by marked irritability and the infant's inability to be satisfied. This clinical picture is often confused with "colic" and may result in frequent formula changes or alterations in breast feeding. In fact, this pattern is often the first "soft sign" that neurological abnormality exits, and will call for changing the approach in handling, positioning, and managing the child.

As the child grows, the oral development problems may involve inability to chew and swallow solids, or to drink from a cup. Complicated multiple deficits in taste of the tongue and proprioception of tongue, lips, and jaw may all play a part. Limitations in head, neck, and trunk control may further limit maintenance of the upright posture in sitting which will affect the infant's ability to participate actively in the feeding process [9].

Abnormality in development of speech itself relates to hearing, intelligence, development of receptive and expressive language, integration of motor mechanisms of the tongue, palate, lips, and associated musculature. Maturation of the breathing pattern from initially nasopharyngeal to predominantly abdominal in the young infant, to thoracic in the normally developing child, may also be impaired and affect the speech mechanism [10].

Thus a fixed central nervous system lesion may influence all areas of oral development through direct effect on the structures of the oral cavity itself as well as indirectly through abnormality of tone, reflexes, and motor behavior involving head and neck. The major consequence is again a restriction of normal active experience with the mouth, its relation to other parts of the body, and to the surrounding environment. As in other areas already discussed, the net effect is to place the child at an experiential disadvantage; to make him or her a passive participant; and to compel a role of dependency. In this sense the neurological lesion serves to entrap such children to "fix" them at an immature stage where they may remain unless some active intervention process alters their relation to the environment.

DEVELOPING AN ASSESSMENT PROCEDURE
OF FUNCTION AND DEFICIT

Determining the appropriate diagnosis and description of neurological deficits provides only one dimension in understanding the meaning of developmental disability. The functional consequences outlined above provide a perspective which must also be considered in achieving an accurate understanding of the child's needs and future requirements. As well as a systematic examination of the neurological and appropriate developmental signs, a thorough investigation of functional limitations must be made as a basis for determining the future course of action.

The starting point is a detailed evaluation of tone, reflex behavior, motor and sensory status, and posture conducted by the therapist upon referral following diagnosis. A procedure which we utilize will be outlined in detail in Chapters 4 and 6. In addition, a transdisciplinary team approach is essential to evaluate the sensory modalities such as vision and hearing, speech, social and emotional status, cognition, and the family situation [11].

For neonates and younger infants, particular attention should be given to problems in management arising out of the deficits identified in the evaluations. For example, hypotonia will have obvious consequences for posture, movement, and motor development. It will also affect many aspects of daily care and management of the child with which the parent will require direct assistance and guidance. Implications for contact with the environment and learning must be given equal consideration.

Management evaluation should cover at least the followng major areas:

1. Handling
2. Positioning
3. Daily care
4. Bathing
5. Dressing
6. Feeding

Handling the child refers to awareness of special requirements for carrying the child, for adequate support, and supervision necessitated by abnormalities of tone, reflex behavior, or motor limitations. Various postures may exaggerate abnormal tone or accentuate immature reflex patterns, for example. Others may enable the child to assume a more physiologic pattern yet be consistent with the tasks required of the parent, and need to be emphasized.

Positioning is similar but relates to specific adaptations that may be necessary in order to deal with the child. What is the best position given the specific limitations for cleaning, bathing, dressing, or feeding? The individual needs will determine how these can best be accomplished so as not to limit further nor tend toward regression of the level of development.

Daily care includes all of the demands for infant management which are made more stringent when the child is developmentally delayed. Physical organization of equipment and space is a first consideration with special attention needed for adaptations of crib, high chair, layette, bathing equipment, and so on [12]. Where there are problems of positioning and handling, the parent must be aware of steps which can be taken in preparation for care and of how the child can be helped to be a more secure participant.

Bathing is a good example of a daily activity requiring special handling and positioning for the infant. Without adequate preparation the child may be totally unstable for support and sitting in a wash basin or tub, which could lead to increase in tone and exaggeration of startle or other primitive reflexes. Moreover, under these circumstances, a potential opportunity for positive contact with the environment and learning could be totally lost. Instead, with stabilization of the child from behind, and emphasis on a midline position, a secure upright posture can be obtained with comfort and freedom of the arms and trunk, allowing the child to participate actively in what can be a productive learning and socializing experience.

Dressing, similarly, is an essential activity with many opportunities for interaction between parent and child, and with the environment. Problems of abnormal tone and pathologic reflex activity, for example, could totally influence the effect of this activity. Specific attention to details of abnormal function involving positioning, handling, and movement patterns as dressing is performed, will enable guidelines to be formulated to deal best with the dressing experience. As with other areas of management a guiding principle should be to assist the child to a secure position so that the youngster can observe and participate actively, if possible, in the entire process. It may involve, for example, obtaining supported sitting with the child being guided from behind in putting on articles of clothing [13]. Functional evaluation must provide an insight into the child's specific deficits which have to be considered in working toward this goal.

Feeding is the child's most complex functional activity. It directly incorporates problems of tone, posture, motor abnormality, and reflex behavior with the head and oral mechanism. As with other areas of management, specific associated abnormalities must be identified as they relate to the feeding process. Here too, the goal is to afford a positive, active experience for the child, to enable ease of care, as well as maximize potential for learning and social development [14]. Specific management and treatment techniques concerned with feeding are reviewed in detail in Chapter 7.

Assessment findings concerning existing deficits, functional needs, and recommendations for continuing care should then be reviewed by the team. In deciding how best to approach the child, consideration must be given to family resources and capabilities, availability of facilities and staff, and a projection of short- and long-range needs.

REFERRAL FOR MANAGEMENT AND THERAPY

Overview of Therapy Methods

Definitive approaches to therapy for the young child with cerebral palsy have
been evolving since the initial attempts of Jennie Colby. The trend toward
very early diagnosis and intervention has greatly shifted initial emphasis away
from orthopedic surgery and placed major priority on global remediation of
the existing developmental deficits and much more emphasis on cognitive
needs. The physical therapy modalities in current use reflect a continuum of
approaches which have evolved over the past 50 years or more for some and
more recently for others. Unequivocal superiority of a given method, including the most recently evolved, has yet to be fully established by adequate
follow-up studies. However, the general relevance of the therapies and early
intervention in affecting significant developmental change is becoming increasingly well-documented [15] (see Chap. 10). The following schools of
therapy are among those which have had the greatest influence on treatment
programs.

Crothers

While not a unique treatment procedure in itself, the approach of Crothers
remains a basic guide to involving the patient in a meaningful program and is
implicit in many of the current acceptable methods [16]. He stressed the
need for active movement and stimulation activities to prevent contractures
and encourage participation, even in the most severely involved children. He
also counseled against overprotection, to enable the child to be more independent and active. Considered truisms today, these tenets offered a new and
comprehensive approach which included the need for individualized assessment following which the child could be realistically directed to appropriate
activities.

Phelps

This method used an orthopedic approach with conventional techniques from
poliomyelitis treatment regimens. Therapy of individual muscles was
stressed. Emphasis also was placed on training in gross movement patterns
and inhibition of abnormal movements. Deep massage was employed for
muscle stimulation. Auditory and kinesthetic activities were used, particularly
a combination of rhymes and music together with desired movement patterns, to develop a conditioned reflex [17]. Once the association was estab-

lished between a musical rhyme and movement, the child was expected to perform the movement upon hearing or reciting the rhyme.

Phelps encouraged visual stimulation with eye-hand coordination activities. Particular stress was placed on the use of orthotic devices for regulation of tone and postural adjustment. Relaxation techniques were used for dyskinesias, synergistic movement patterns were used, namely, resisting one muscle group, to achieve movement in synergy. For example, he provided resistance to hip flexors in order to activate foot dorsiflexors.

Weights were highly regarded in treatment of ataxia. Stretching exercises were advocated for spasticity, with a heavy emphasis on the use of full control braces. The goal would be to reduce the extent of bracing as control was achieved about a particular joint.

In many respects, Phelps was the first to develop a coherent systematic approach. Much of his teaching remains in active use today in some form.

Deaver

Deaver emphasized functional ability rather than patterns of movement. His objectives included [18]:

1. Performance of bed and wheelchair activities
2. Maximum use of hands
3. Performance of ambulation and stair climbing
4. Achievement of adequate speech and hearing
5. Achievement of as near normal appearance as possible

The method employed extensive bracing, restricting all but two movements of an extremity in functional activity. Reduction in extent of bracing would occur as functional control was achieved.

Considerable emphasis was placed on intensive training as well as in activities of daily living (ADL), particularly wheel chair use [19]. For this purpose, periods of treatment were prescribed to take place in a residential unit, at frequent intervals as the child developed and needed to acquire new skills for function. Finally, surgery was often recommended for cosmetic reasons alone, such as to improve wrist flexion, or provide ankle stabilization, even when functional change would not be expected.

Fay-Doman

Fay, a neurophysiologist, early postulated the concept of motor developmental levels of the brain comparable to the evolutionary process [20]. The most primitive levels relate to the lowest forms and development progresses through maturation at each level. Thus the brain must evolve through stages of fish, and reptile, for example, finally toward mammalian species and ultimately humans. This highly controversial concept is frequently expressed as "ontogeny recapitulates phylogeny," or development of the individual recapitulates evolution of the species [21]. An insult or injury to the central nervous system interrupts this process with fixation at a given lower or immature stage. Thus, the child with anoxia is fixed at a primitive stage from which he or she cannot appropriately evolve as homosapiens without an induced process which mirrors the suggested evolutionary brain process.

Doman, a trained physical therapist, took these concepts and integrated them into a system of therapy commonly referred to as "patterning." In this system, a child must become proficient at each level before going on to the next [22]. The child is placed in prone position, using various ipsilateral and contralateral patterns of head turning and arm and leg movements. Graded developmental stages are used progressively including crawling, creeping, and walking with cross patterns.

Ancillary stimulatory procedures may be used simultaneously such as inhalation of carbon dioxide and use of deep pain with pin pricks. Fluid restriction was also suggested to reduce cerebrospinal fluid pressure [23].

The patterning procedure is practiced on a regular daily schedule, usually using four or more volunteers for each administration. Parents are intimately involved in organizing and following the treatment process and meet with professionals at regular intervals for assessment of progress and assignment of a new treatment schedule. This is a highly controversial theory and method. Demands upon both child and family are severe. Positive results are considered by many to be questionable; harmful effects likely to be common and extensive [24]. It is not recommended by a number of medical and surgical subspecialties [25].

Rood

Both sensory and motor aspects of movement received equal emphasis in this system. The basis lies in activating muscles through sensory receptors, and then using a sequence of developmental patterns of movement [26]. The emphasis is on developing an early awareness of normal patterns since it is obviously more difficult to correct abnormal patterns later.

Sensory receptor stimulation is accomplished by applying heat or cold accompanied by stroking or brushing of selected areas along a muscle group. Heat is particularly used for relaxation. Selection of stroking or brushing would depend upon the muscle groups involved, degree of tension, or restriction, and response to stimulation. Developmental patterns of movement are then encouraged to achieve physiological function with reinforcement.

Kabat-Knott

These procedures utilize facilitation mechanisms to increase voluntary muscle contraction through central excitation. Exercises use large movement patterns to activate and strengthen weak muscles. Mass movements are also used to simulate normal functional activities. A variety of spiral and diagonal movements are also part of this "proprioceptive neuromuscular facilitation" which generally requires a cooperative and well-motiviated patient [27].

Bobath and Neurodevelopmental Therapy (NDT)

The Bobaths have had the most recent and perhaps most extensive influence in the therapy field. Their treatment system is a neurodevelopmental approach to the total underlying deficits that relate to tone, movement, and posture. The basic abnormality is considered to be impairment of primitive and postural reflexes associated with abnormal tone. By extension there will be developmental deficits of posture, movement, and progression in motor maturation [28].

The approach is to evaluate thoroughly the state of reflex development, and its effect on tone, posture, and movement. Treatment centers around inhibtion of abnormal reflexes to alter tone, and facilitation procedures of reflex behavior to develop normal patterns of posture and movement [29]. The system has been subject to changes in emphasis and direction and continues to be flexible in its approach to understanding the total underlying neurological maturation mechanism.

The wide appeal of Bobath NDT therapy has led to extensive training programs for therapists throughout Europe and the United States. Certification in neuro-development treatment (NDT) has gained considerable status as a mark of professional expertise in this field and is sometimes implied to be the only recognized professional training for those working with children.

Recently, the entire concept of abnormal reflex behavior has been questioned by Milani-Comparetti [30], who found increasing evidence from intrauterine studies which suggests that reflexes are operative long before birth and continue to be present on a lifetime continuum. He suggests that stimulation and eliciting of "reflexes" leads to a response which is neither normal nor abnormal, but appropriate for that individual. He further questions a therapy approach based on "abnormal" reflexes. Whether this criticism can alter or influence the treatment approach remains to be determined.

Others

Vojta. This method emphasizes a preventive approach and attempts early identification of infants at risk for cerebral palsy [31]. Criteria for abnormality utilize deviation from a number of postural reflexes, primitive reflexes, and asymmetries. The treatment procedure involves early reflex creeping and turning procedures before 6 months of age [32]. While popular in some parts of Europe and in Japan, the method has not gained acceptance in the United States.

Peto. Emphasis is away from the approach of individual therapy treatment and stresses global integrated management. The method is based on a conductive educational approach and abolishes the traditional division of treatment into specific therapies and replaces it with a unified approach and a single therapist who acts as the "conductor." Integration of many simultaneous sensory-motor-cognitive activities is stressed in group treatment settings [33,34]. Basically, the method is practiced in Hungary and other parts of Europe and has recently gained considerable popularity.

In overview, it can be said that in the United States there has been a virtual withering away of the practice of most individual systems of therapy as we knew them 20 years ago.

One sees very little evidence of reliance today upon a conditioned approach such as Phelps, Deaver's exclusive use of bracing; the concepts of sensory stimulation in Rood; or large muscle therapy of Knott. There does indeed continue to be a strong emphasis on the facilitation techniques of Bobath now referred to as neurodevelopmental therapy. What this approach clearly has given us is a global developmental method of both evaluating and viewing progress in a child and structuring the goals that are to be achieved. It has moved us away from concentration upon limitations in a particular joint or functional disability, and enabled us to place the child on a scale of development so that his needs could be better assessed and approached.

Eclectic Approach. In the clinical situation today many knowledgeable therapists use an eclectic approach. They first thoroughly evaluate the total patient (deficits and needs), both for management and stimulating treatment. They then may choose a variety of modalities from several of the established schools of therapy as the basis of treatment. This selective approach offers great flexibility and gives the therapist an opportunity to tailor to the child's needs as well as the professional's capabilities and interests. No particular term is given to what is the most frequently employed method. Its advantages are easily recognized. However, an obvious disadvantage relates to its lack of uniformity and systematization which offers difficulty in evaluating and comparing results. This could be overcome by more exact description and identification of the procedures followed.

Therapy in Relation to Other Accepted Treatment Modalities

Early Intervention Programs

Treatment of cerebral palsy by definition must deal with the developmental needs of a multiply handicapped child. The areas of disability go far beyond motor development and maturation alone. Moreover, there are finite limitations to what can practically be expected of therapy programs as the child grows and develops. Therapy can be offered as the earliest approach to treatment but is now among many available modalities which have been shown by experience to be acceptable for the complex needs of the growing child [35]. Moreover, emphasis has now shifted from a concentration on individual systems of treatment to widespread programs of early intervention which incorporate physical, occupational and speech therapy, with infant/childhood development, and early education methods. How these programs further develop and are used, and in what relationships remains a matter of judgment and clinical experience, as well as availability.

Medication

The use of drugs to alter the motor deficit of cerebral palsy and improve movement has a relatively recent and generally unsuccessful history. Their use with infants and young children has usually been limited to patients in at least the later preschool years. A variety of muscle relaxants have been tried with little benefit [36].

Dantrolene sodium also has generated conflicting claims of benefits and may be associated with serious liver dysfunction [37,38]. It use in childhood cerebral palsy has not been demonstrated to be effective. However, in the stroke patient with a hemiplegia it has shown evidence of some functional effect [39].

Tranquilizers, such as chlordiazepoxide and diazepam, have been used with some effect in relief of increased tone and movement in the athetoid child [40]. In conjunction with an active therapy program, these are considered by some to be a useful and a temporary adjunct in the total approach to the child [41]. As with all of the drugs used, none presently offers effective and sustained relief from motor, tone, and postural deficits by itself.

L-dopa had been used in the athetoid patient with some conflicting results [42,43]. Generally, some early response was noted, but long-term effects are not seen [44] and side effects often cannot be tolerated.

With respect to the major associated handicaps, however, drugs do play a significant and often mandatory role. Anticonvulsants are essential in management of seizure disorders and must be continuously reevaluated. Where indicated, medication for attention deficit disorder and hyperactive behavior, especially in the older child, is required to obtain maximum participation. Drug treatment for the severely emotionally disturbed child also has a place and may be a primary consideration before specific therapy for the cerebral palsy can take place.

Orthotic Devices and Equipment

A variety of functional aides are available for therapy programs for the infant and very young child. The prone or supine board, corner chair, feeding chair, other adaptive seating arrangements, sensory and motor stimulating toys, and specialized feeding equipment are a few of the many innovations that both therapist and parent can use to deal with individual requirements. Such equipment is increasingly being devised with an awareness of its potential value in motor development and teaching. Considerably less emphasis is now being placed on use of standing tables and other rigid essentially passive structural and devices merely to contain the child.

Bracing in cerebral palsy has a long history and was often employed as the definitive modality. Its use as a treatment procedure in itself is now not accepted since experience has shown it to be often restrictive, passive, and generally without active carryover unless as part of an active therapy program. In conjunction with orthopedic surgery procedures, however, it has a well-established place to maintain position and improve function.

Use of braces together with a therapy program has both proponents and detractors. Bracing is generally discouraged for the infant and very young child with generalized cerebral palsy, with the emphasis on therapy to help achieve head control, sitting, and initial weight bearing. With growth and persistent functional dependence, many clinicians would consider offering some form of brace for the lower extremities in the hope of overcoming deforming forces and stablizing posture and gait. Therapy and bracing then need not be exclusive but may be mutually supplemental in helping to achieve functional development. It should be kept in mind that bracing has a definite effect on sensation as well as motor functioning. Also the use of braces should be task oriented—for example in standing or weight bearing. Functional orientation will enable better integration into the overall therapy program.

The child with an obvious early hemiplegia might be considered a suitable candidate for short-leg bracing at a very young age to prevent contracture and enable earlier weight bearing. Again, there need not be conflict with a therapy program if functional goals are clear.

As the child develops toward weight bearing and ambulation, appropriate use and progression to walkers, crutches, and canes must be carefully considered. In addition, shoe inserts may be very useful in improving foot deformity and stabilizing gait. Wheelchairs are also becoming more functional and many types are now available which offer better maneuverability and ease of handling, together with better controlability of the child. With active involvement in a therapy program there is less concern about dependency on introducing a wheelchair early, especially if it forms part of a functional treatment program.

Surgery

Neurosurgery. Surgical correction of any brain lesion associated with cerebral palsy in the infant would involve treatment of hydrocephalus, possible vascular anomalies, cysts, or benign tumors. Intractible seizures may respond to partial resection of brain tissue or even hemispherectomy in highly selective cases [45]. Obviously if any of these conditions are a serious consideration, appropriate identification and surgical management is mandatory and has priority over any other treatment considerations.

The procedure of chronic cerebellar stimulation had been offered in the past. This utilizes an implanted electrical pacemaker to reduce tone, control extrinsic movement, and increase function primarily in adults with cerebral palsy [46]. Limited effectiveness over a prolonged period and possible significant placebo response were frequent [47]. This procedure has not generally been used with infants. It remains an area of investigative neurophysiologic engineering and has not become an established modality.

A recent procedure which has gained considerable attention is selective posterior rhizotomy [48]. The procedure identifies and then divides nerve rootlets associated with an abnormal motor response following lumbar laminectomy. Left intact are rootlets associated with a brief localized contraction. Definite reduction in spasticity and improved tone is reported in selective cases. Sustained or long-term effects are yet to be clarified or results replicated. Whatever the outcome, it is clear that the procedure would have no effect on abnormal CNS integration in cerebral palsy.

Orthopedic care and management have a major role in very early treatment of cerebral palsy. In conjunction with other medical specialists and therapy staff, the orthopedist provides guidance and direction in conservative approaches to limit or prevent abnormality and use of special equipment.

As the child grows and maximum benefit is obtained from therapy, bracing, and other conservative measures, orthopedic surgical procedures may be considered to overcome residual deformity and improve function. The judgment of when and how extensively to operate is the key to proper orthopedic care. Early and continuous involvement with the child provides the best hope for the most realistic and appropriate surgical intervention.

Corrective eye surgery for strabismus should be performed as early as appropriate to prevent amblyopia. *Repair of cleft lip and then palate* is similarly essential in the very young child. Other types of corrective procedure may be necessary and could be planned in conjunction with the continuing therapy program.

Behavior Modification

This is a positive reward system to stimulate new or alter previous behavior with roots in psychology [49]. A specialized aspect, biofeedback, involves voluntary change affecting physiological parameters such as blood pressure or heart rate [50]. Data from the psychology literature confirm effectiveness of the technique for many discrete types of behaviors, especially for short time periods [51]. It has been utilized in the preschool child in gait training to overcome equinus [52], and in the infant to improve head control and sitting [53]. Planning the target behavior and developing the reward or reinforcement procedure requires a joint effort of therapist and psychologist. Sometimes the procedure can be used to condition the child to the therapy session itself to obtain a better cooperation and participation.

The technique may have much to offer in a broader way than presently recognized and deserves wider application. For example, its use in dealing with self-abusive or other unacceptable social behaviors is increasingly apparent [54]. This type of behavior may be seen in children with various levels of mental retardation and organic brain deficits. It can greatly affect management both in the home, therapy, or school situations and referral for an appropriate behavior management program should be considered part of the total multidisciplinary approach which can be offered.

Social and Mental Health Services

A major advantage of working with the affected infant is that it provides the opportunity of becoming totally involved with the family. Often the child is identified only after a period of diagnostic confusion and a long search for the appropriate agency. Anxiety and guilt are frequently felt by the family. Conflicting information and advice about care or treatment may be overwhelming. Physical problems concerning finances and transportation may prevent needed participation. These and other problems require an active social service program with involvement in the home when needed. Counseling and definitive psychiatric referral and care must also be available. Parental discussion groups in conjunction with the therapy program can offer the support and direction to assure carryover at home and an atmosphere conducive to growth. Professionals should not lose sight of the fact that appropriate support and care at home is the major ingredient reported by older patients, in long-term follow-up studies, to have influenced their functioning and development [55].

Special Education

Early intervention programs for cerebral palsy and other developmental disabilities are proliferating within the United States and throughout the Western world. The models vary considerably; some are home-based and totally individualized, others utilize group methods with therapists and educational specialists. These often offer the earliest form of special education for the child and a new form of special education for the parent. Whenever possible, the therapy program should be integrated into such a total educational effort enabling contact with other infants and families. This can greatly influence early learning and social maturity of the child, and provide the support and direction needed by families.

Recent extension of the Education for All Handicap Act of 1975 (P.L. 94-142) now mandates the provision of appropriate preschool programs for children from 3 to 5 years (P.L. 99-457) [56]. Of particular interest is the fact that this legislation also has an "enabling" feature now allowing provision for educational programs as well up to age 3 in school districts throughout the United States. (See Chap. 9 concerning evaluation of both therapy and early intervention—education programs.)

Controversial Treatments

Management and treatment programs clearly require use of a variety of modalities. Timing, emphasis, and application will vary with the strengths and orientation of professionals, and as a result programs will differ. This is a natural consequence of continual change in technology, experience, and results of outcome.

Some procedures are in use and may have appeal yet are strongly questioned because of methods employed or outcomes claimed. This is true for patterning therapy (Fay-Doman) which is strongly criticized and not recommended for referral by the major medical specialty societies [25,57].

The neurosurgical procedure of chronic cerebellar stimulation is considered experimental in nature with little established benefit noted on long-term follow up. Results with the new approach of dorsal rhizotomy are also yet to be clearly well established.

Hypnosis has been used with older children [58], and acupuncture has also been advocated without any evidence of meaningful benefit [59]. Optometric exercises are widely prescribed for perceptural motor deficits, coordination, and balance, but long-term effects are difficult to evaluate [60]. Diet therapy is commonly employed for behavioral and perceptual problems, including the Feingold regime and use of megavitamins. The former area in particular is now being closely scrutinized for possible relevance [61,62]. Vestibular stimulation has been studied in a control design and was found to have no significant effect [63] although Chee et al. had previously shown positive results [64].

A field dealing with chronic disability always requires the search for new and better approaches. It is hoped that a basic principle of objective evaluation and relevance to existing treatment will be kept in mind.

Developing the Prescription for Evaluation and Therapy

Identification of the child with significant developmental delay or with a definite diagnosis of cerebral palsy should lead to referral for appropriate care without delay. The physician and other professionals should be familiar with relevant resources within the community which can provide needed services, or at least be able to refer the patient to a source of information. The present evidence supporting early evaluation and intervention will be helpful in obtaining parental understanding and acceptance. Professional direction in finding the appropriate resource can help avoid "shopping" among agencies, ensure good communication, and avoid unnecessary delay in treatment. It is also essential that, following referral, the physician maintain active contact with the treatment agency to enable close follow-up of the patient and guidance for the family.

The referral for therapy is essentially a prescription and should include the basis for concern, diagnosis, and need for further work-up, and specific functional evaluation. These requests should first consider management problems to assist the family with care of the child. A full examination of sensory and motor development would then be expected so that the child can be placed in an appropriate treatment program. The elements of *management and treatment* should both be included in the prescription to ensure the most appropriate planning for the abnormally developing child.

Generally, the local medical society will have a listing of agencies offering services for the young child. State offices of United Cerebral Palsy can be contacted for location of local chapters where more information can be obtained. Easter Seal and similar other local agencies can provide information on relevant programs.

REFERENCES

1. Zapella, M. The blink reflex to light in the newborn: Relation to light evoked cortical potentials in the EEG. *Dev. Med. Child. Neurol.* 9:287, 1967.

2. Vlach, V., Bermuth, H. von, and Prechtl, H. State dependency of exteroceptive skin reflexes in newborn infants. *Dev. Med. Child. Neurol.* 11:353, 1969.

3. Graziani, L., Weitzman, E., and Velasco, M. Neurological maturation and auditory evoked responses in low birth weight infants. *Pediatrics* 41: 483, 1968.

4. Cavins, G., and Butterfield, E. Assessing infant's auditory functioning. In Friedlander, B. et al. (Eds.): Exceptional Infant, Vol. III. New York, Brunner, Mazel, 1973, pp. 84-108.

5. Ingram, T. Clinical significance of the infantile feeding reflexes. *Dev. Med. Child. Neurol.* 4:159, 1962.

6. Logan, W., and Bosma, J. Oral and pharyngeal disphagia in infancy. *Pediatr. Clin. North Am.* 14:47, 1967.

7. Brown, J. Feeding reflexes in infancy. *Dev. Med. Child. Neurol.* 11: 641, 1969.

8. Bosma, F. (Ed.). Second Symposium on Oral Sensation and Perception. Springfield, Charles C Thomas, 1970.

9. Adran, G., and Kemp, F. Some important factors in the assessment of oropharyngeal function. *Dev. Med. Child. Neurol.* 12:158, 1970.

10. Cook, C., Lucey, J., Drorbaugh, J., Segal, S., Sutherland, J., and Smith, C. Apnea and respiratory distress in the newborn infant. *N. Engl. J. Med.* 254:562, 1956.

11. Haynes, U. A Developmental Approach to Case Finding with Special Reference to Cerebral Palsy, Mental Retardation, and Mental Disorders. Washington, D.C., Public Health Service Publication No. 2017, 1970.

12. Finnie, N. Handling the Young Cerebral Palsied Child at Home, London, William Heinemann, 1976.

13. Connor, F., Williamson, G., and Siepp, J. (Eds). Program Guide for Infants and Toddlers with Neuromotor and Other Developmental Disabilities. New York, Teachers' College Press, 1978.

14. Sholl, C., and Scherzer, A. Feeding problems of the cerebral palsied infant. *Pediatr. Dig.* 16:19, 1974.

15. Tjossem, T. (Ed.). Intervention Strategies for High Risk Infants and Young Children. Baltimore, University Park Press, 1976.

16. Crothers, B. Disorders of the Nervous System in Childhood. New York, Appleton, 1926.

17. Phelps, W. The rehabilitation of cerebral palsy. *South. Med. J.* 34:770, 1941.

18. Deaver, G. Methods of treating the neuromuscular disabilities. *Arch. Phys. Med. Rehabil.* 37:363, 1956.

19. Deaver, G. Cerebral Palsy: Methods of Evaluation and Treatment. Rehabilitation Monograph IX. New York, Institute for Rehabilitation Medicine, 1952.

20. Fay, T. The use of pathological and unlocking reflexes in the rehabilitation of spastics. *Am. J. Phys. Med.* 33:347, 1954.

21. Gould, S. Ontogeny and Phylogeny. Cambridge, Harvard University Press, 1977.

22. Doman, R., Spitz, E., Zucman, E., Delacato, C., and Doman, G. Children with severe brain injuries. Neurological organization in terms of mobility. *JAMA* 174:257, 1960.

23. Gilette, H. Systems of Therapy in Cerebral Palsy. Springfield, Charles C Thomas, 1969.

24. Cohen, H., Birch, H., Taft, L. Some considerations for evaluating the Doman-Delacato "patterning" method. *Pediatrics* 45:302, 1970.

25. American Academy of Pediatrics, Policy statement: The Doman-Delacato treatment of neurologically handicapped children. *Pediatrics* 70:810, 1982.

26. Rood, M. Neurophysiological mechanisms utilized in the treatment of neuromuscular dysfunction. *Am. J. Occup. Ther.* 10:4, 1956.

27. Knott, M., and Voss, D. Proprioceptive Neuromuscular Facilitation, Patterns and Techniques. New York, Hoeber, 1963.

28. Bobath, K., and Bobath, B. The facilitation of normal postural reactions and movements in the treatment of cerebral palsy. *Physiotherapy* 50:246, 1964.

29. Bobath, K., and Bobath, B. Cerebral Palsy. In Pearson, P. (Ed.), Physical Therapy in the Developmental Disabilities. Springfield, Charles C Thomas, 1972, pp. 31-185.

30. Milani-Comparetti, A. Fetal movements and cerebral palsy—a new classification. San Francisco, American Academy for Cerebral Palsy and Developmental Medicine, 1979.

31. Brandt, S., Lonstrup, H., Marner, T., Rump, K., Selmar, P., and Schack, L. Prevention of cerebral palsy in motor risk infants by treatment ad modum Vojta. *Acta Paediatrica Scand.* 69:283, 1980.

32. d'Avignon, M., Noren, L., and Arman, R. Early physiotherapy and modum Vojta or Bobath in infants with suspected neuromotor disturbance. *Neuropediatrics* 12:232, 1981.

33. Cotton, E., and Parnwell, M. From Hungary—The Peto method. *Spec. Educ.* 56:7, 1967.

34. Cottam, P., McCartney, E., and Cullen, C. The effectiveness of conducive education principles with profoundly retarded multiple handicapped children. *Br. J. Dis. Commun.* 20:45, 1985.

35. Silver, L. Acceptable and controversial approaches to treating the child with learning disabilities. *Pediatrics* 55:406, 1975.

36. Denhoff, E. Drugs in Cerebral Palsy. Little Club Clinics in Developmental Medicine. London, Heinemann, 1964.

37. Herman, R., Mayer, N., and Mecomber, S. Clinical pharmaco-physiology of dantrolene sodium. *Am. J. Phys. Med.* 51:296, 1972.

38. Chyatte, S., Birdsong, J., and Roberson, D. Dantrolene sodium in athetoid cerebral palsy. *Arch. Phys. Med. Rehabil.* 54:365, 1973.

39. Mayer, N., Mecomber, S., and Herman, R. Treatment of spasticity with dantrolene sodium. *Am. J. Phys. Med.* 52:18, 1973.

40. Keats, S., Morgese, A., and Nordlund, T. The role of diazepam in the comprehensive treatment of cerebral palsied children. *Western Med. J.* 4:22, 1963.

41. Denhoff, E. Cerebral palsy—pharmacologic approach. *Clin. Pharmacol. Ther.* 5:947, 1964.

42. Rosenthal, R., McDowell, F., and Cooper, W. Levodopa therapy in athetoid cerebral palsy: a preliminary report. *Neurology* 22:1, 1972.

43. Goodman, A., Goodman, L., and Gilman, A. The Pharmacological Basis of Therapeutics. New York, MacMillan, 1980, p. 487.

44. McDowell, F., Lee, J., and Sweet, R. Extrapyramidal Disease. In Baker, A., and Baker, L. (Eds.), Clinical Neurology. New York, Harper and Row, 1978, vol. 2, p. 49.

45. Davidson, S., Falconer, M., and Stroud, C. The place of surgery in the treatment of epilepsy in childhood and adolescence. *Dev. Med. Child. Neurol.* 14:796, 1972.

46. Cooper, I., Riklan, M., Amin, I., Waltz, J., and Cullinan, T. Chronic cerebellar stimulation in cerebral palsy. *Neurology* 26:744, 1976.

47. Medical News. Chronic cerebellar stimulation. *JAMA* 242:315, 1979.

48. Peacock, W., Arens, L., and Berman, B. Cerebral palsy spasticity. Selective posterior rhizotomy. *Pediatr. Neurosci.* 13:61, 1987.

49. Bandura, A. Principles of Behavior Modification. New York, Holt, Rinehart and Winston, 1969.

50. Green, E., Green, A., and Walters, E. Voluntary control of internal states: psychological and physiological. *J. Trans. Pers. Psychol.* 2:1, 1970.

51. Hawkins, R., Peterson, R., Schweid, E., and Bijou, S. Behavior therapy in the home. Amelioration of problem parent-child relations with the parent in a therapeutic role. *J. Exp. Psychol.* 4:99, 1966.

52. Block, J., and Silverstein, L. Integrating biofeedback-bioengineering approaches into a comprehensive cerebral palsy treatment center. New Orleans, American Congress of Rehabilitation Medicine, 1978.

53. Silverstein, L. Biofeedback with young cerebral palsy children. In Feingold, B., and Bank, D. (Eds.), Developmental Disabilities of Early Childhood. Springfield, Charles C Thomas, 1978, pp. 142-147.

54. McGee, J. Bonding as pedagogical phenomenon—A data based analysis of how children and adults with severe behavioral problems learn to interest with their care givers. Cathleen Lyle Murray Lecture. American Academy for Cerebral Palsy and Developmental Medicine. Boston, 1987.

55. Symposium: People with cerebral palsy talk for themselves. New York American Academy for Cerebral Palsy, 1971.

56. American Academy of Pediatrics. Committee on Children with Disabilities: Pediatrician's role in development and implementation of an individual education plan. *Pediatrics* 80:750, 1987.

57. Freeman, R. Controversy over "patterning" as a treatment of brain damage in children. *JAMA* 202:385, 1967.

58. Nieburgs, T., Goldenson, R., Nieburg, H., and Kline, M. Hypnotic approaches to neuromuscular impairment: speech rehabilitation of the cerebral palsied: Atlanta, American Academy for Cerebral Palsy and Developmental Medicine, 1977.

59. Spears, C. New approach to treatment of cerebral palsy: auricular therapy (acupuncture). Atlanta, American Academy for Cerebral Palsy and Developmental Medicine, 1977.

60. American Academy of Pediatrics. Joint organizational statement: The eye and learning disabilities. *Pediatrics* 49:454, 1972.

61. Conners, C., Goyette, C., Southwick, D., Lees, J., and Andrulonis, P. additives and hyperkinesis: A controlled double-blind experiment. *Pediatrics* 58:154, 1976.

62. American Academy of Pediatrics, Committee on Nutrition. Megavitamin therapy for childhood psychoses and learning disabilities. *Pediatrics* 58:910, 1976.

63. Sellick, K., and Over, R. Effects of vestibular stimulation on motor development of cerebral palsied children. *Dev. Med. Child. Neurol.* 22:476, 1980.

64. Chee, F., Kreutzberg, J., and Clark, D. Semicircular canal stimulation in cerebral palsied children. *Phys. Ther.* 58:1071, 1978.

4

Normal and Abnormal Sensorimotor Development

OVERVIEW

The infant who is given a diagnosis of cerebral palsy by the pediatrician or neurologist is referred to physical, occupational, and speech therapy for further assessment and for treatment. The growing availability of early intervention programs allows referrals to therapy to be made as early as possible and preferably before subtle signs turn into marked symptoms upon which a positive diagnosis of central nervous system (CNS) dysfunction can be made.

At this point, the infant has undergone a developmental evaluation as described in Chapter 2. A more detailed qualitative assessment of sensorimotor functions is now in place. Thorough knowledge of normal and abnormal development is a prerequisite for such a detailed assessment.

A model for general principles of sensorimotor development is presented and applied to the course of normal as well as abnormal development. Implications of abnormal postural and oral development are discussed. Motor behavior is analyzed more specifically as to the underlying postural reflex mechanism and to intrinsic motor components which determine quality of postural alignment (function of righting reactions) and the degree of balance (function of equilibrium reactions). Using illustrations, components of various abnormal movement patterns are contrasted with normal responses. The interaction between various movement components is described.

With CNS impairment, important components of posture and movement fail to develop. The infant is ill-prepared for subsequent developmental skills and more and more abnormal responses are perpetuated. Sensorimotor behavior, when seen in a truly developmental sense, can be interpreted as the summation of preceding experiences as well as a preparation for future motor skills. Abnormal components of movement, even when subtle, can have alarming significance as potential obstacles to normal sensorimotor development.

GENERALIZED CONCEPTS OF SENSORIMOTOR DEVELOPMENT

NORMAL DEVELOPMENT

Research points to the presence of vast prenatal experiences in motor activity and sensation of movements. Fetal movements display an organization into clearly defined motor patterns [1,2], and the repertoire of postnatal movements and motor activities seems to be mostly a reflection and continuation of fetal motor patterns.

The neonate, although often described as functioning on a reflex level, is nevertheless equipped with a sizable variability of motor patterns. However, the postural control against gravity is very limited during the first weeks and months of life. The first year in particular, and to a substantial part the following four to five years are dedicated to the acquisition of this postural control and balance. The automatic responses mostly responsible for this control are the righting and equilibrium reactions and other components of the postural reflex mechanism.*

The development of postural control proceeds generally in a cephalo to caudal direction as well as in a proximal to distal direction. The infant first acquires postural control and balance of the head before trunk balance and, finally, the ability to control movements of the pelvis and legs. Similarly, postural stability of the shoulder girdle, for example, prepares the development of skillful hand functions. However, the development of postural control should not be divided arbitrarily; and the interplay between cephalo to caudal and proximal to distal occurs in both directions. For example, head control can be refined only on the basis of some trunk control and shoulder girdle stability.

Postural control must occur in three planes, but development of this three-dimensional control seems to follow a specific sequence.

Plane 1 Achieves control in the *sagittal plane* with the use of extension as well as flexion against gravity. Postural organization in the other planes

---

*For a detailed discussion on the development of the postural reflex mechanism see Chap. 9.

is limited to cephalocaudal weight shift (transverse plane) and maintaining symmetry (frontal plane).

Plane 2 Control in the *frontal plane* is completed when lateral righting and balance of asymmetrical postures are established.

Plane 3 Postural control in the *transverse plane* is fully mastered through rotation within body axis.

There is, of course, a smooth and overlapping transition between these stages.

This sequence is repeated at different positional levels, namely first in prone and supine, then in sitting, crawling, and, finally, in standing and walking. It is interesting to correlate this pattern to the sequential development of movement direction in visual skills, in eye-hand coordination, and in the percept-concept formation. There, the sequence generally progresses also from the vertical to the horizontal to the diagonal direction, as for example, in building with cubes or in drawing.

A general pattern can, furthermore, be observed in the development of postural control of extension against gravity before postural control of flexion against gravity. The initial pattern of extension allows the infant to move out of a pattern of physiological flexion. Extension is then modified and graded through the counterbalance of flexion as a function of mature reciprocal inhibition. Again, this sequence occurs in the different positions.

The extremities move from a mostly flexed posture which is exhibited by the neonate toward extension and abduction before full extension and adduction is established. Rotation is, again, the last component the infant learns to grade.

During the course of development, a progression can be seen from total motor synergies to dissociated or differentiated motor patterns. Initially, any action encompasses the whole body. Gradually, the infant learns to move one part of the body independently from other body parts and, furthermore, starts to combine components of different motor patterns, such as patterns of flexion and extension. Although some isolated movements can already be seen in the neonate, these are random. A persistent and purposeful application of selective, isolated and fine-tuned motor acts requires a high degree of inhibitory control, in other words, inhibition of total and excessive movements, and develops in accordance with the progressive maturation of the brain.

ABNORMAL DEVELOPMENT

Abnormal sensorimotor development may start in utero and the subsequent postnatal development of some infants may be a continuation of abnormal fetal sensorimotor experiences.

Early abnormal development is frequently expressed in exaggerated reflex behavior with a simultaneous absence of variability and adaptability of responses. Some reflexes may also be suppressed and weak, as for example, some of the feeding reflexes. In contrast with normal development where primitive reflex behavior gradually decreases while righting and equilibrium reactions emerge, primitive reflexes are not modified in cerebral palsy and may be used for function when more adaptive responses such as righting and equilibrium reactions fail to develop.

Most often, however, sensorimotor deficits are not detected during the very first weeks or months of life. The symptoms of clearly abnormal motor reactions appear later and especially when the infant attempts to assume more upright positions. Without intervention, the severity of the symptoms increases during the course of development, although the brain lesion itself is stable and not progressive in cerebral palsy. Emerging abnormal motor patterns can be seen as a combination of neurological and kinesiological factors.

Abnormal development also proceeds generally in a cephalo to caudal direction and, depending on the distribution of impairment, initial symptoms usually occur in the area of head control and trunk control, while posture and movements of the legs may still appear normal. Also, abnormal distal movement components usually can be traced back to abnormal proximal movements.

Sequential development of postural control for the three planes of the body is often arrested at the initial phase. Patterns of extension and flexion dominate the motor behavior, while lateral righting is often delayed and rotation within the body axis is impaired.

Patterns of extension frequently predominate and are not graded by a flexor component. Due to this disturbed reciprocal innervation, the antigravity extension differs not only in quality and grading but also in distribution (see Motor Patterns at Different Developmental Stages and Postural Control in Prone). Postural control of flexion against gravity is often poorly developed.

The last postural component of the limbs which emerges in a spastic pattern is the rotation. This is comparable to the sequencing in normal development. The abnormal extensor pattern, for example, is expressed initially in pronounced extensor tonus followed by progressive adduction and finally by internal rotation.

Central nervous system (CNS) dysfunction is expressed as a lack of inhibitory control. As a result, differentiated and selective movements cannot be executed. Instead, total and synergic motor patterns continue to characterize the motor behavior.

MOTOR PATTERNS AT DIFFERENT DEVELOPMENTAL STAGES

To identify a delay in development, it is important to know sequencing and timing of developmental milestones. There exists a vast literature on normal development. A selection of publications on this topic is included in the bibliography. To identify abnormal sensorimotor development as seen in cerebral palsy, it is necessary to analyze motor patterns and movement components which make developmental milestones possible. The analysis of motor patterns described in this chapter is based mostly on clinical experience [3-6].

MOTOR PATTERNS OF HEAD CONTROL

NORMAL

Postural control against gravity develops with the influence of righting reactions which brings the head into proper position in space. Some degree of head control is first displayed in supported upright and in prone positions (Fig. 1a). Newborns are already able to extend the neck and to lift the head

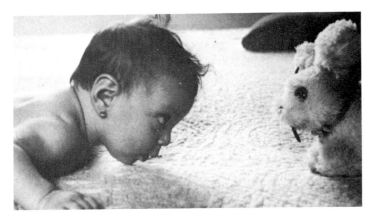

Figure 1a (Normal). In prone, early head control is achieved through extension of the head (atlanto-occipital joint) and the spine (cervical and upper thoracic) bringing the face to a 45 degree angle toward the support (2 months). (Photograph by Christine Nelson.)

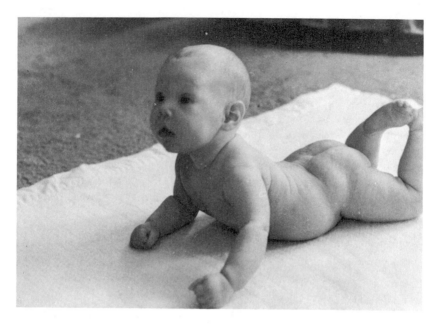

Figure 1b (Normal). Mature head righting indicates a fine interplay between extension and flexion. This brings the face into a vertical and the mouth into a horizontal position while elongating the neck. Free head movments can occur on a stable spine (4 months).

briefly to free the nasal pathways while lying prone. At approximately 4 months of age, this primitive form of extension is altered with the integration of a flexor component allowing the infant to tuck the chin in and maintain the face in a truly vertical plane. With the activation of pectorales muscles (flexor component), the infant pushes up on the elbows with more accent than before. The shoulders broaden and the neck elongates (Fig. 1b). Gradually, the baby learns to dissociate head movements from movements of shoulder girdle and trunk.

The ability to raise the head in supine comes somewhat later (by about

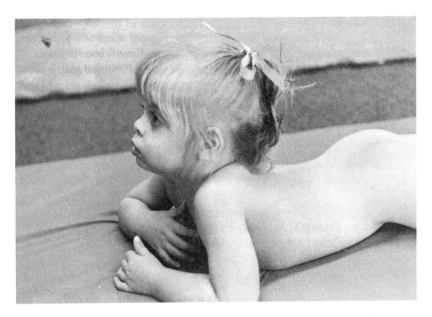

Figure 2 (Abnormal). Hypotonicity and poor coordination between flexion and extension lead this girl to raise her head with hyperextension of head and neck. Poor trunk stability interferes with free head and arm movements. Compare with Fig. 1b.

5 months). From then on the head is well-balanced in all positions. In upright positions the same posture appears as in prone. The combined activation of extension and flexion keeps the face in a vertical plane and elongates the neck.

ABNORMAL

Primitive posture. In abnormal development, the head posture is frequently affected. The primitive pattern of hyperextension of head and neck persists. Shoulder elevation usually accompanies this posture (Fig. 2). Head and shoulders move as one unit. This posture is basically seen in all positions.

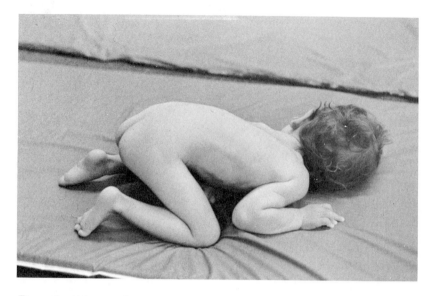

Figure 3 (Abnormal). Abnormal progravity flexor tonus causes this infant to weight bear on her head while in prone. Raising the head is therefore inhibited.

Abnormal flexor tonus. In prone position, abnormal flexor tonus may pull the infant into gravity. In this case the weight of the body rests on the head and the arms, similar to the newborn. As a result, raising the head and the development of normal extensor patterns throughout the body are severely restricted (Fig. 3).

Abnormal extensor tonus and asymmetry. Efforts to move or to raise the head may result in extensor hypertonicity throughout the body. Predominant extensor patterns encourage asymmetry. Asymmetry of head posture may result in asymmetry throughout the body, especially when the influence of the asymmetrical tonic neck reflex (ATNR) is strong. Persistent reinforcement of this asymmetry interferes with the very important stage of symmetry

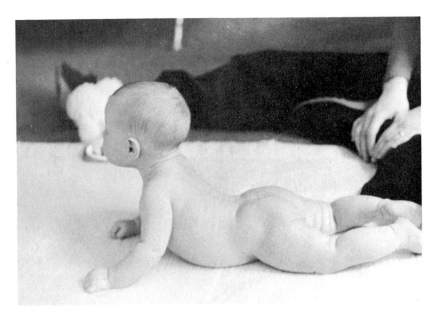

Figure 4 (Normal). The "chain reaction" of extension against gravity requires coordination between axial extensors and flexors (abdominals, extensors of spine and hips) to enable the infant to stabilize the pelvis and to raise head and chest off the support (5 months). Observe, there is little weight on the arms due to good spinal stability.

and midline orientation. An asymmetrical head posture can also be seen in the hemiplegic child who orients toward the less impaired side. Rotation of the head is combined with lateral flexion to the skull side and with shoulder elevation.

POSTURAL CONTROL IN PRONE

NORMAL

Head lifting in prone starts a "chain reaction" of extension against gravity (Fig. 4). Complete antigravity extension is expressed in the Landau reaction,

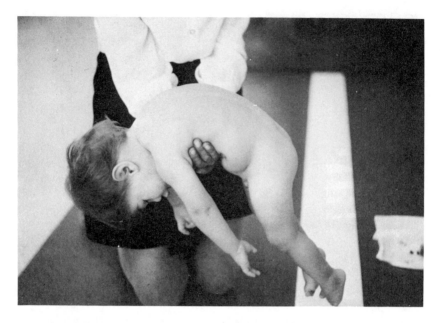

Figure 5 (Abnormal). Hypotonicity is especially obvious in ventral suspension. Head righting and extension against gravity are lacking. Some hypertonicity is obvious in the pattern of adduction and internal rotation of the hips and plantarflexion of the feet. (From *The Infant with Cerebral Palsy: An Approach to Identification, Management and Treatment*, A. L. Scherzer. Private printing, New York, 1973.)

which is attained between 5 and 8 months and which can be observed first in prone ("swimming" posture, prone on hands), and subsequently in ventral suspension. In the "swimming" posture, axial extension is combined and reinforced with scapular adduction and retraction in the shoulder joint. This motor pattern reappears later in the "high guard" posture in sitting, standing, and walking as a transient phase before better postural control and balance are developed. In the Landau reaction, neck and trunk extend and the legs assume a pattern of extension, slight abduction and external rotation of the hips, extension of the knees and, mostly, dorsiflexion of the ankles. A strong

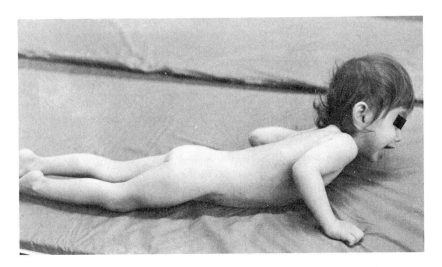

Figure 6 (Abnormal). Abnormal extensor tonus limits extension against gravity and results also in abnormal posturing of the limbs, such as adduction and internal rotation of the hips and extension of the shoulders. Compare with Fig. 4.

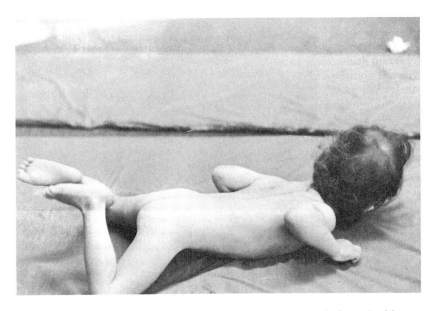

Figure 7 (Abnormal). When axial extension is not counterbalanced with flexion, the pelvis is pulled off the support and the body weight rests to a great part on the chest. The asymmetry of the head posture also indicates lack of flexor control. Compare with Fig. 1b.

Landau reaction also provides the infant with some form of locomotion, for example, by propelling backward on extended arms.

Complete antigravity extension can develop only when postural stability is allowed through the counterbalance of flexion. To raise head and chest off the support, the pelvis needs to be stabilized as a point of support to move against. Abdominal action and subsequent hip extension are required to stabilize the pelvis. Extension of the hips makes it possible to bring the legs closer together, which facilitates weight shifting to one side. The weight shift promotes the amphibian reaction with dissociation of movements between the two sides of the body. This leads to controlled rolling, crawling, and creeping.

ABNORMAL

Abnormal postural tonus. Extension against gravity may be suppressed by abnormal flexor tonus which pulls the infant into gravity when in prone (see Fig. 3). Very low postural tonus also restrains righting against gravity (Fig. 5). The effort to move against gravity may reinforce the development of extensor hypertonicity which is especially obvious in the posturing of the legs: adduction of the hips and plantar flexion of the ankles. Later on, internal rotation of the hips emerges. Although the legs are extended, the hips cannot fully extend due to the anterior pelvic tilt (Fig. 6). This pattern differs distinctly from the Landau reaction.

Poor integration between extension and flexion. When integration between flexion and extension is disturbed, proper righting against gravity cannot develop. In prone, the pelvis cannot be stabilized against the support and active hip extension is therefore not possible. As a result, weight bearing cannot shift down to the pelvis (Fig. 7).

Primitive flexor pattern of the legs. A pronounced pattern of hip flexion and abduction ("frog posture") interferes with the chain reaction of extension against gravity. This also interferes with weight shift and locks the infant into a static posture.

POSTURAL CONTROL IN SUPINE

NORMAL

Although they display a flexed posture, neonates lack controlled flexion against gravity. During the first few months, extension activity increases, not only in prone but also in the supine position. The limbs, which were initially positioned close to the body, move gradually into more extension and abduction. The increasing extensor tonus reinforces an asymmetrical posture which is highlighted in the ATNR attitude. This is most pronounced during the second month of life. A month later, active flexion against gravity permits the infant to keep and control the head in midline. Until then a sustained midline position of the head occurs predominantly during sucking and crying. Midline orientation of the head occasions postural symmetry throughout the body (Fig. 8a). The eyes start to converge, the hands come together, and bilateral movements of the limbs dominate.

Midline orientation and flexion against gravity permit investigation of the body. The eyes focus on the hands during play or while the infant reaches toward the legs. With more flexor control, the legs can be raised against a stable trunk and pelvis which brings the feet into the visual field and into the range of manual and oral investigation. With a combination of flexion and extension patterns the infant raises the extremities with extended knees and elbows. While holding on to the legs the infant rocks from side to side, vigorously exercising the abdominal muscles during the performance of differentiated balance reactions (Fig. 8b).

Integration between flexion and extension can also be seen in the postural alignment of the spine. The whole back rests on the support while the infant lies in supine. Integration between flexion and extension soon leads to new movement components such as lateral righting of the trunk, axial rotation, and differentiated movements of the limbs. These new movement components enable the infant to move out of the supine position (Fig. 9).

ABNORMAL

Postural asymmetry. Postural asymmetry persists when reciprocal innervation between flexion and extension does not mature. This is especially pronounced in the ATNR posture and causes lateral curvature of the spine and torsion of pelvis and trunk, especially when the ATNR influence is predominantly to one side. Lateral hiking and forward rotation of the pelvis on the skull side lead in time to adduction and internal rotation of the hip which is then in danger of luxation (Fig. 10).

Hypertonicity. Extensor hypertonicity results in hyperlordosis of the cervical and lumbar spine. As a consequence, the pelvis is tilted anteriorly and the hips are in some degree of flexion. Arms and shoulder girdle are retracted (Fig. 11). Excessive flexor tonus seems to be mostly a secondary problem.

Lack of antigravity tonus. Flexion against gravity develops poorly when hypotonicity prevails. These infants usually assume a flexed and widely ab-

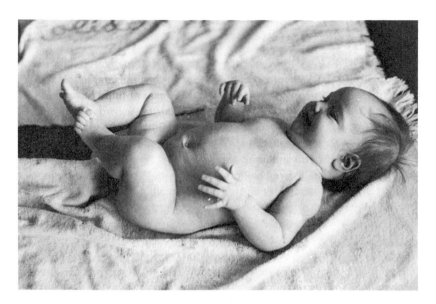

Figure 8a (Normal). The development of flexion against gravity is necessary for sustained midline orientation of the head which produces a symmetrical posture throughout the body (3 months).

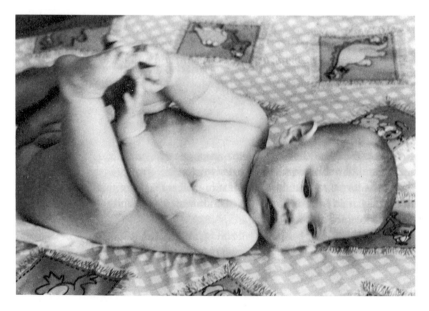

Figure 8b (Normal). Stronger flexor control enables the infant to move the legs on a stable pelvis high enough for the feet to be reached and to be in the visual field. Lateral weight shift and crossing of midline elicit balance reactions as a direct preparation for balancing in longleg sitting (5 to 6 months).

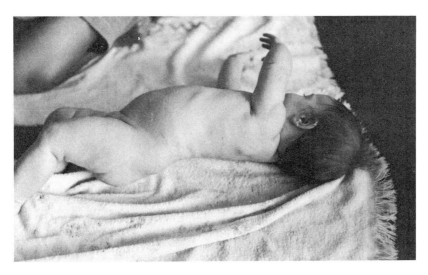

Figure 9 (Normal). Initial attempts of rolling from supine to side are initiated mostly by pushing into extension. Nevertheless, posture of head and arms indicates control of both, extension and flexion (4 months).

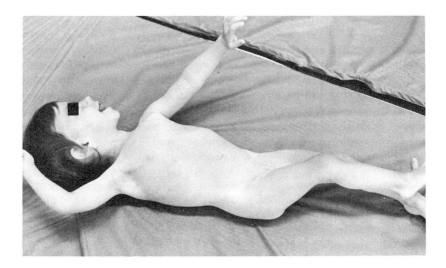

Figure 10 (Abnormal). A dominating influence of tonic reflexes (ATNR) pulls the right arm and shoulder back when the head is turned toward the left. As a consequence, this girl is unable to move out of supine. The pelvis rotates in the same direction as the head. Adduction and internal rotation of the right hip is a further component of this associated pattern. Compare with Fig. 9.

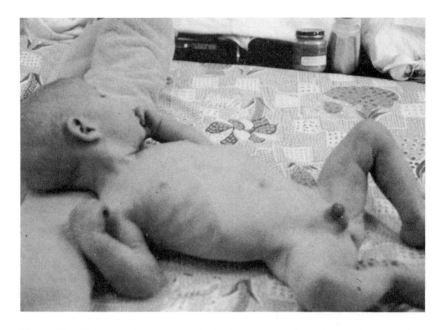

Figure 11 (Abnormal). Turning of the head, retraction of shoulders and arms as well as the wide abduction of the hips ("frog" posture) indicate lack of flexor control and suggest extensor hypertonicity. Compare configuration of chest and abdomen with Fig. 8a. (Photograph by Christine Nelson.)

ducted posture of the limbs. The broad bilateral abduction interferes with weight shifting and does not permit a change of position. While these infants initially sink into gravity, they may, later on, develop extensor hypertonicity.

Lack of sustained antigravity tonus, severely hampers body investigation and bilateral hand play. The hypotonic infant when able to raise the feet off the support does so with marked abduction and flexion of the hips. Without abdominal action, trunk and pelvis are not stabilized, and legs and feet cannot be brought into the visual field. Control of the extremities in space is not practiced.

Some infants learn to use extension for bridging and even for some form of progression. In contrast with the normal pattern, the extension occurs predominantly in the spine with little active participation of the hip extensors. Ungraded extension is also used for rolling and, of course, cannot provide good movement control nor appropriate righting against gravity.

PATTERNS OF UPPER EXTREMITY WEIGHT BEARING

NORMAL

The newborn already bears weight on the arms when lying in prone. The majority of the body weight rests on chest and head and the ulnar side of the hand and arm. During the first month, the posture of the arms changes so that the weight bearing occurs on the palmar side of the hand (which is usually slightly fisted) and on the ventral side of the forearm. (Grasping is initiated also on the ulnar side of the hand, progressing to a palmar and, finally, to a radial grasp.) Gradually the arms move further away from the body into more abduction and the elbows are finally placed in vertical alignment with the shoulders (by about 3 months). This corrects the posture of scapular protraction and permits the development of independent head movements. With increasing balance between patterns of flexion and extension, the elbows move closer together into shoulder adduction allowing the infant to shift weight laterally when prone on forearms (by about 4 months) (Fig. 12a).

Increased extension activity of the upper trunk leads to increasing scapular adduction. Antigravity adduction of scapulae is most pronounced in the "swimming" posture which is exhibited in prone by about 5 months. Yet, in normal development, this strong extensor phase is offset by the forward-reaching in supine.

Dissociated movements between trunk, scapula, and humerus develop specifically during weight shifting in prone posture. These movements are important for the development of a dynamic shoulder girdle on a stable trunk preparing for more accurate reaching and providing a stable base for controlled head movements. Lateral righting and movements of the trunk against the weight bearing arm are also practiced in the side position (Fig. 12b,c).

In addition to weight bearing, visual and oral investigation of the hands as it occurs mostly in supine position, prepare for the development of manipulative skills. When infants first reach toward objects, they overshoot their movements and require considerable practice in reaching objects accurately, especially when the hand is positioned out of the visual field (5 to 6 months).

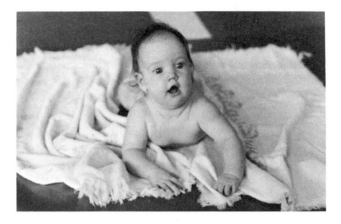

Figure 12a (Normal). Vertical alignment between shoulder and elbow enable the infant to develop balancing in prone on forearms and to maintain the alignment between head and shoulder girdle during lateral weight shift (3 to 4 months).

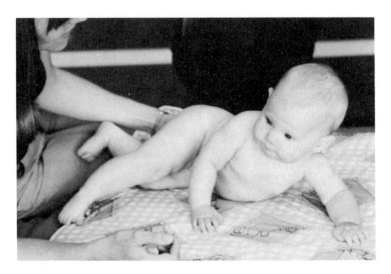

Figure 12b (Normal). Lateral control is challenged to a greater degree in the side position. Lateral head righting elicits the amphibian reaction, causing elongation on the weight-bearing and lateral flexion on the non-weight-bearing side. The pattern of the right foot provides positional stability (6 months).

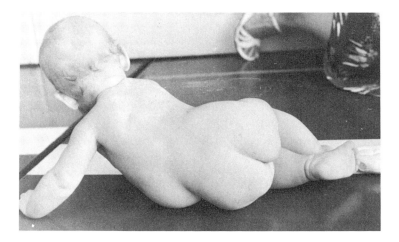

Figure 12c (Normal). Play activities in side propping require good shoulder girdle stability. Rotation within body axis is achieved by rotating the weight-bearing shoulder back and/or by rotating the contralateral hip back (8 months).

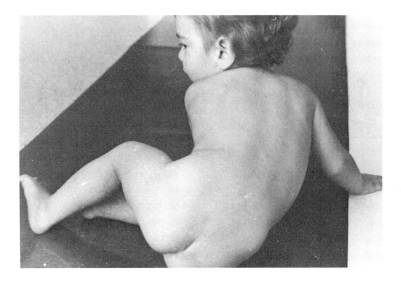

Figure 13 (Abnormal). Scapular protraction occurs as a compensation for poor trunk stability, interfering with axial rotation and balancing. Compare with Fig. 12c.

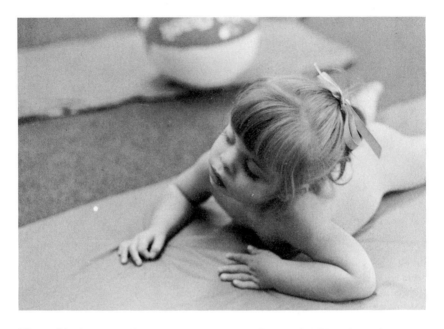

Figure 14 (Abnormal). A primitive pattern of wide shoulder abduction provides some postural stability but interferes with a balanced lateral weight shift. Instead of shifting the weight through the lower trunk and the pelvis, this girl tilts the head toward the weight-bearing side. As a consequence, lateral righting is not elicited.

ABNORMAL

Scapular protraction. In abnormally developing children, primitive patterns of weight bearing are often retained. In prone position, extension of the shoulders causes the hands to be placed caudally in relation to the shoulders which encourages scapular protraction while restricting free head movements. Scapular protraction causes internal rotation and pronation of the arm, especially when combined with shoulder abduction. Internal rotation of the arms interferes with proper weight bearing on the hands. The weight rests mostly on the radial side of the hands. The hands are often fisted and may be positioned in ulnar wrist deviation. Strong internal rotation can result in weight bearing on the dorsum of the hand. Consistent scapular protraction is combined with excessive flexion of the thoracic spine. As a consequence, head and trunk balance cannot fully develop. Intrinsic trunk movements such as rotation between shoulder girdle and pelvis cannot take place (Fig. 13).

Proximal stability. Coordination between patterns of extension and flexion is needed for a stable spine and to stabilize the scapula on the trunk while the arm moves. Infants with poor reciprocal innervation compensate for lack of stability with wide shoulder abduction. For lateral weight shift, the head is tilted which negates proper righting of head and trunk (Fig. 14).

Associated movements of scapula and humerus. Extension of the thoracic spine reinforces scapular retraction and shoulder extension. This "W" position of the arms is typical for the pure extensor pattern during early phases of abnormal development. The same posture appears at different stages of normal development and has been called "high guard." There it accompanies initial phases of independent sitting, standing, and walking before appropriate proximal control emerges. However, in a more stable position the normal infant moves out of the high guard posturing. In abnormal development this posture is maintained in all positions and the infant does not learn to move scapula and humerus independently, but continues to move them as one unit. In time, the mobility between scapula and humerus is drastically decreased and leads to excessive winging of the scapula whenever the arm is moved. Scapular stability cannot develop. Impaired shoulder girdle stability is a consequence of poor stability of the spine. Head movements, accurate reaching, and fine graded manipulative skills are impeded.

POSTURAL CONTROL IN SITTING

NORMAL

Infants sit square on their buttocks, with the pelvis perpendicular. However, due to lack of extension against gravity the babies demonstrate a rounded back in supported sitting up to about 3 months of age. From then on, extension progresses gradually in a cephalo to caudal direction (Fig. 15). When infants start briefly to sit unassisted, the lumbar spine is still rounded (5 to 6 months of age). To ensure balance, infants may prop themselves on the hands or may hold both arms in the "high guard" position. By that time, the infant has developed head balance but not full trunk balance in sitting. Head right-

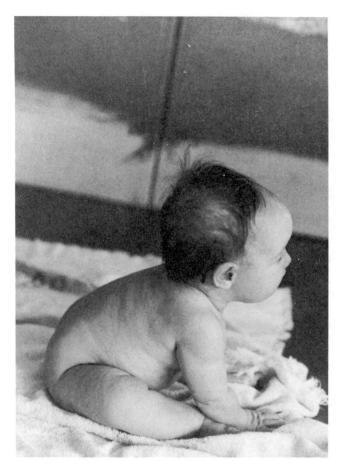

Figure 15 (Normal). Before extensor control of low back and hips develop fully, the infant leans forward in sitting. The legs are positioned in a total flexor pattern providing a broad base of support (3 to 4 months).

ing facilitates trunk righting (Fig. 16). Coordinated activation of extensors and flexors of trunk and hips must be achieved before equilibrium reactions emerge somewhat later in sitting [by about 8 months (Fig. 17)]. Trunk movements can by then be better differentiated from movements of pelvis and legs. This permits, for example, flexion of hips combined with full extension of the lumbar spine. This improved trunk balance is expressed in a more narrow base of support, for example, the legs are no longer in a primitive and total flexor pattern but are brought closer together and extended at the knees. Secure sitting balance enables the infant to assume a variety of sitting postures. Furthermore, appropriate trunk control frees the hands for manipulation in sitting (Fig. 18). Preceding and partially overlapping with the emergence of equilibrium is the development of protective extension of the arms (Fig. 19).

Balance in one position is only fully developed when the infant is able to assume the position or move out of it in a controlled fashion. During the early months of life the infant cannot effectively assist when pulled to a sitting position, and by 4 months head control is sufficiently developed so that the infant can keep both the head and trunk in alignment when pulled to sitting (Fig. 20). With increased stability of shoulder girdle and trunk the 5- to 6-month-old infant can actively pull up when hands are held. Attempts to get to sitting independently are first successful from the prone position (7 months). Later the infant rolls from supine to side lying and pushes up to sitting with the arms (10 months), while the symmetrical way of sitting up from supine is achieved much later (by 5 to 6 years).

ABNORMAL

Lack of extension against gravity. A flexed sitting posture, where the trunk falls forward into gravity, is typical in many hypotonic infants. The degree of flexion is exaggerated even in comparison with the normal neonate. At the same time, the head may "hang back" in hyperextension (Fig. 21).

Excessive extension. Some infants demonstrate premature and abnormal extension of the spine with a "high guard" posture of the arms. By leaning the trunk forward relative to the vertical line, these infants compensate for the lack of pelvic control. Wide abduction of hips provides positional stability and allows the pelvis to tilt forward (Fig. 22).

In other cases, abnormal extension may also be seen in the posture of the legs. Extensor hypertonicity leads to adduction at the hips and plantarflexion at the ankles. Later on, internal rotation of the hips emerges as a final component of the abnormal extensor pattern.

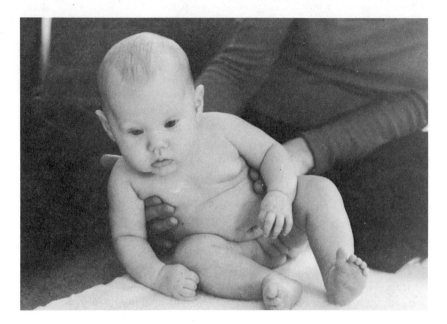

Figure 16 (Normal). When the center of gravity is displaced laterally, righting reactions ensure proper alignment of the head in space. The lateral flexion of the head elicits lateral flexion of the trunk and increased abduction of the limbs on the non-weight-bearing side (5 months).

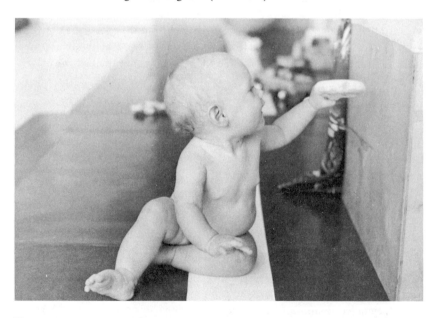

Figure 17 (Normal). Dissociation of movement between trunk, pelvis and hip allows a variety of balanced sitting postures (8 months).

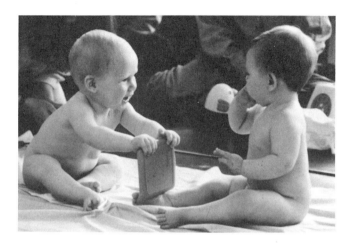

Figure 18 (Normal). Increased trunk control allows free manipulation of toys in unsupported longleg sitting. Control and mobility of pelvis and hips enable the infant to sit with pelvis and trunk in an upright position, to extend the knees and bring the legs close together (8 to 10 months).

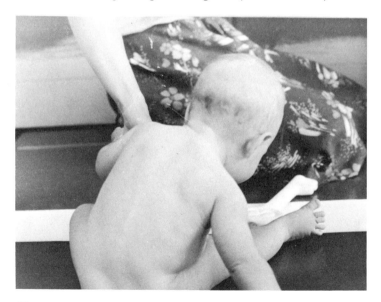

Figure 19 (Normal). When the center of gravity is displaced diagonally backward, the infant reacts with trunk rotation and with protective extension of the arms backward (10 to 12'months).

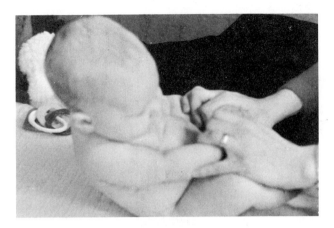

Figure 20 (Normal). Flexor control against gravity enables the infant to align head and trunk when pulled to sitting. Head flexion results in flexion throughout the body, including a total flexor pattern of the legs (5 months).

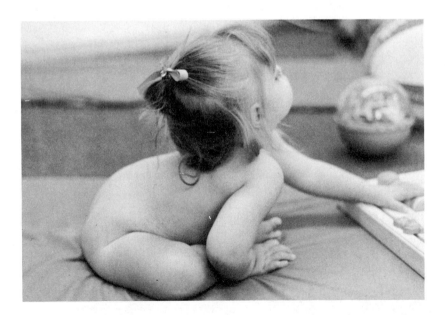

Figure 21 (Abnormal). Flexion of hips and lower trunk are excessive due to hypotonicity which causes this infant to collapse into gravity. Hyperextension of head and neck limit her visual interaction with the toy. Compare with Fig. 15.

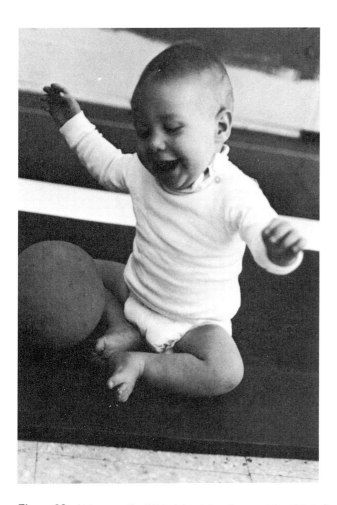

Figure 22 (Abnormal). Wide hip abduction enables this infant to maintain some stability in compensation for impaired control of trunk and pelvis. Compare with Fig. 18.

Compensatory flexion. The initial abnormal patterns demonstrated in prone and supine (see Postural Control in Prone, Postural Control in Supine) are often altered when the infant assumes a more upright position, such as sitting. Compensatory flexion of the upper trunk, neck, shoulder girdle, and arms

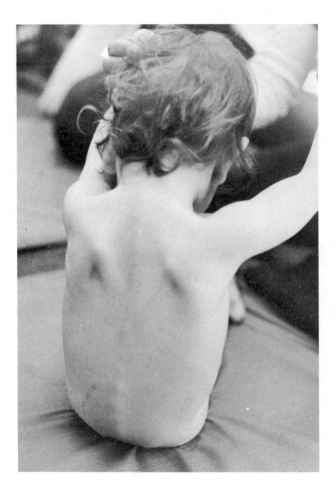

Figure 23 (Abnormal). Tight hip and back extensors pull the pelvis back to a degree where the infant sits on the sacrum. Poor coordination between extensors and flexors prevents an upright posture of pelvis and trunk. Compare with Fig. 18.

may be superimposed on the early, ungraded extensor patterns present in lower positions. Furthermore, head and mandible may be thrust forward. This occurs specifically when the extensors of the lower back and hips are shortened and, therefore, pull the pelvis back in longleg sitting. Contrary to

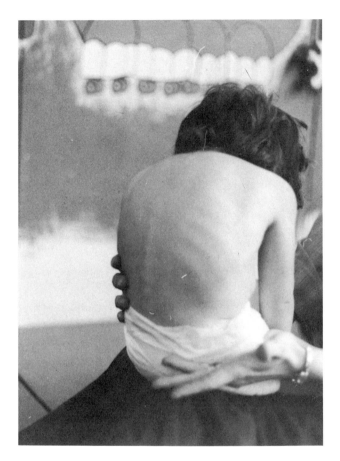

Figure 24 (Abnormal). Pronounced flexion of the upper trunk may develop as an attempt to bring the center of gravity forward over the base of support. Flexor spasticity may increase as a consequence which can lead to structural deformities.

normal infants, these infants sit on the sacrum (Fig. 23). Head, arms, and upper trunk are brought forward to gain some balance. For the infant to see the surroundings, the head must be tilted back. When an infant spends lengthy periods in this sitting posture the compensatory flexion may increase flexor spasticity and may modify primary motor patterns in lower positions (Fig. 24).

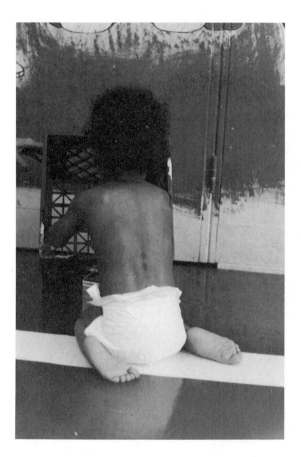

Figure 25 (Abnormal). Sitting between the heels ("W"-sitting) compensates for lack of mobility and balance, and allows vertical alignment of pelvis and trunk. The broad base of support discourages any lateral or diagonal weight shift resulting in a very static posture. Asymmetry of weight bearing is common (see hips and feet). Consistent adduction and internal rotation of the hips affect further development of the lower extremities.

To compensate for lack of mobility and balance the handicapped infant often assumes the "W" sitting position: sitting between the heels, which provides a broad and stable base. This is a very static posture which does not promote any weight shifting or the development of trunk and pelvic control (Fig. 25).

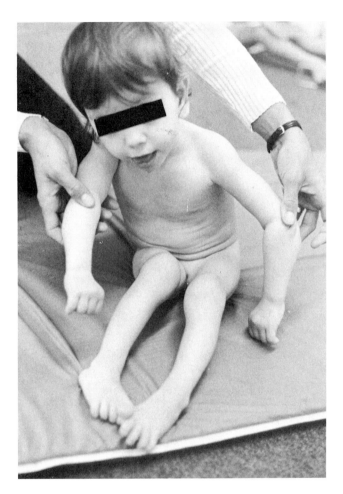

Figure 26 (Abnormal). Association of motor patterns results in retraction of trunk and pelvis. Alignment and balance are severely impaired.

Asymmetry of weight bearing. Predominant asymmetry of the pelvic posture is abnormal. It affects postural alignment throughout the body and patterns of weight bearing. Balance is threatened (Fig. 26). Some infants learn to sit unsupported by using head and upper trunk for balancing or by leaning on the hands, but in such a position, activities are limited.

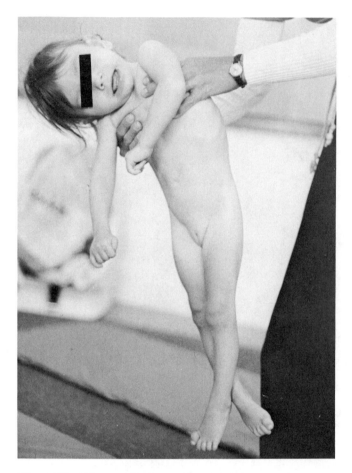

Figure 27 (Abnormal). Lateral head righting can also be tested in vertical suspension. With head and trunk falling into gravity, spatial orientation must be difficult. Compare with Fig. 16.

Impaired righting and equilibrium reactions. None of these sitting postures is conducive to the infant developing good sitting balance. At best compensatory pattern skills are improved, but these compensations are restrictive to further development. While head righting is poorly developed, trunk righting cannot follow (Fig. 27). The poor head and trunk control means that

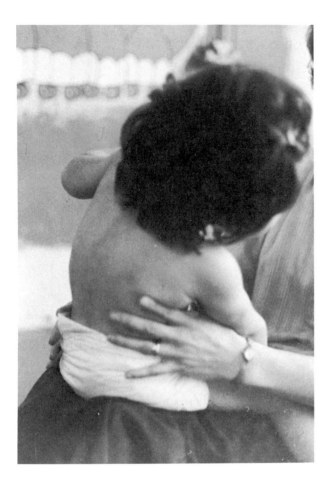

Figure 28 (Abnormal). Abnormal postural tonus and flexion of the upper trunk prevent this girl from rotating her right shoulder back for protective extension of the arm. Compare with Fig. 19.

hands are not free for manipulation, the shoulders are elevated with the scapula either protracted or retracted. All these abnormal compensations are a poor beginning for protective extension of the arms (Fig. 28).

Poor sitting balance is combined with an inability to sit unassisted or move into and out of sitting in a controlled fashion. When the infant is pulled into

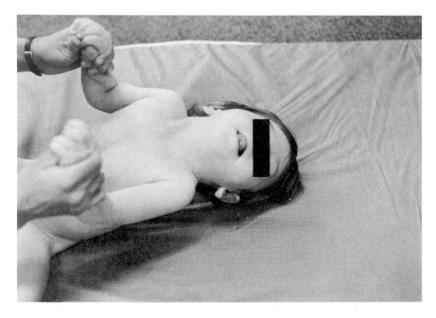

Figure 29 (Abnormal). This child shows severe head lag when pulled to sit. Hypertonicity is also expressed in the oral posture. Compare with Fig. 20.

sitting position, the head drops back and the shoulders elevate, indicating poor integration between axial extension and flexion (Fig. 29).

PATTERNS OF LOCOMOTION

NORMAL

In the prone position, the neonate is capable of some locomotion in the form of "crawling" movements, with symmetrical extension and flexion of the legs. The mature and more efficient pattern of belly crawling, however, differs substantially from this primary crawling and requires more refined postural skills. Similar to any mature form of locomotion, crawling is initiated by a lateral weight shift. Before the infant attempts to crawl, he or she has obtained much practice in lateral weight shift and lateral body righting, as for example, in prone on arms. The lateral righting of the trunk leads to a reaction of the legs, and the infant assumes the posture of the amphibian reaction: elongation and extension on the weight-bearing side, shortening and flexion on the non-weight-bearing side. By about 5 months, the lateral weight shift occurs more and more from the pelvis which causes the pelvis to rotate. This, in turn, permits the infant to pull the knee forward into flexion on the non-weight-bearing side. Now, the infant can push from the knee while both arms pull the body forward (at about 5 to 6 months). Gradually, the foot assists more in this action. First the infant pushes with the medial side of the foot; but soon he or she learns to use the toes to push off more efficiently.

With progressive differentiation of motor patterns, the infant is able to assume the fourpoint-kneeling position. Controlled weight shift is prepared for by rocking movements which, if vigorous enough, may result in the infant pushing the crib around. Initially, the stability in the quadruped postion is ensured through a broad base. The hips are abducted and externally rotated. The back may sway slightly. Creeping in this posture requires little active trunk balance. Trunk rotation is not yet possible in this position. Instead, the pelvis hikes laterally with each step. With the development of trunk rotation and equilibrium reactions in quadruped, the knees are brought closer together (under the body). By about 9 to 10 months reciprocal creeping patterns emerge. Variety of postures in fourpoint crawling indicate increased balancing skills and differentiation (Figs. 30 and 31).

ABNORMAL

The urge for locomotion may be strong in the handicapped infant but too often the child is ill-prepared for the task. Patterns of weight shifting are deficient even in less demanding situations as, for example, in prone on forearms. Head and body righting are incomplete. A tendency toward total motor patterns inhibits the development of differentiated movements such as the amphibian reaction or rotation of trunk and pelvis. Nevertheless, many handicapped infants learn to creep and to crawl, although in an abnormal and less efficient way.

Commando crawling. Due to their poor ability for weight shifting through the pelvis, infants may pull themselves forward exclusively with the arms while on their stomach. The effort involved causes, in time, an increase of

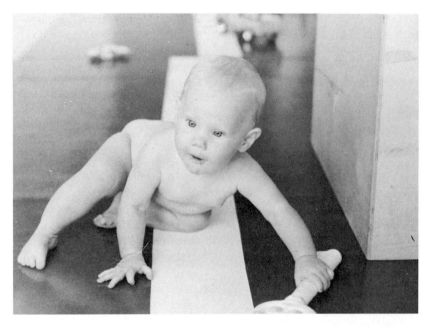

Figure 30 (Normal). Before the infant is able to control rotation within the body axis in the quadruped position, she rotates the leg under the body (flexion, abduction, and external rotation of the hip) while moving toward sitting. A high degree of mobility and dissociation is required for this maneuver (8 months).

extensor hypertonicity of the legs which are totally passive in this action. The legs are then extended although full hip extension is absent due to the anterior pelvic tilt and lumbar hyperlordosis. The hips are pulled more and more into adduction while the feet are plantarflexed (Fig. 32). This is a poor preparation for subsequent standing and walking.

While the weight shift in commando crawling is occasioned almost exclusively through head movements, some infants may learn to shift the weight more through the trunk but in an abnormal way. Using excessive extension, they wiggle and twist pelvis and legs from side to side while the legs are up in the air. The posture of the legs may simulate full hip extension but all the extension actually occurs in the low back.

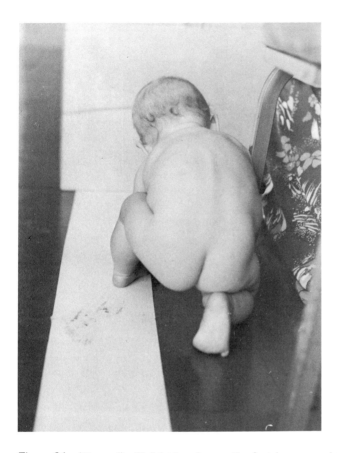

Figure 31 (Normal). Weight bearing on the feet is prepared for in many positions other than standing (see also Figs. 12b and 30). In this posture, the sensory input of weight bearing is reinforced by the infant's sitting on the heel. The right foot is in a state of readiness (push off) for a weight transfer or for a change of position (8 months).

Asymmetry of weight bearing. The infant who uses mostly asymmetrical postures and movements learns to use both limbs (arm and leg) together in belly crawling, but only on one side. The head is turned to the same side and the contralateral side of the body is mostly ignored and "dragged along." In time, increased tightness of the nonactive side results due to associated

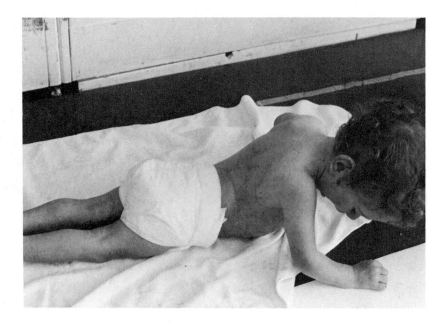

Figure 32 (Abnormal). Commando crawling is a typical form of locomotion in abnormal development. Without lateral weight shift through the pelvis, the legs cannot actively participate and consequently the body is pulled forward with excessive flexion of the arms. The effort involved, increases extensor hypertonicity of the legs.

reactions. Hypertonicity and tightness are expressed in the posture of the trunk (lateral flexion), pelvis (torsion), and extremities (flexion of arm, extension of leg).

Poor proximal stability. When postural control of shoulder girdle, trunk, and pelvis is poorly developed, infants compensate by shifting the center of gravity backward over excessively flexed legs in the quadruped position (Fig. 33a,b). This interferes with lateral weight shift through lower trunk and pelvis. Important patterns of amphibian reaction and axial rotation cannot develop. Lack of dissociation of movements frequently leads to "bunny hopping."

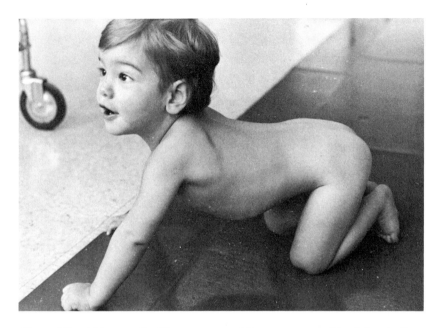

Figure 33a (Abnormal). The pronounced flexor pattern of both legs indicates poor proximal control. Lack of postural refinement leads to weight bearing on the dorsum of the toes. Compare with Fig. 31.

The same abnormal posture of pelvis and legs is used in knee walking and affords a means of progression especially for the athetoid infant who lacks functional upper extremity weight bearing capability. Again, the pelvis is "locked" in a pronounced anterior tilt which inhibits any intrinsic righting and balance reactions of the trunk. Therefore, a change of position can only occur into "W-sitting" which further reinforces a very similar static posture.

Progression in sitting. When strong postural asymmetry is present, fourpoint creeping may be totally omitted. Instead, the infant may learn to propel while sitting by using the arm and leg of the same side as the contralateral side is "dragged along" and ignored, as in belly crawling.

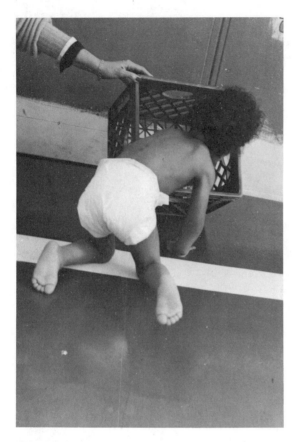

Figure 33b (Abnormal). With increasing hypertonicity the more primitive flexor pattern of the legs changes and the hips pull into adduction and internal rotation. In this position, movements are very restricted. The infant can either "bunny hop" or sit back between the heels (see Fig. 25).

PATTERNS OF STANDING (SUPPORTED, UNSUPPORTED)

NORMAL

The upright posture of standing and walking represents a final stage in the development of postural control against gravity. This process starts with the neonates' instinctive drive to lift the head while prone.

When held in an upright position, the neonate is already capable of supported standing and reflexive walking which are remnants of essential motor acts in utero. During the walking reflex of the full-term infant, the weight is on the whole sole of the foot, and the ankle is in slight dorsiflexion. This early skill soon disappears and emerges later in an altered version as a more controlled gait pattern. During early attempts at supported standing, the center of gravity is not fully aligned over the feet (Fig. 34a). Postural adaptations and movement patterns which infants have acquired in lower positions are practiced again in supported standing. Some of these patterns are: extension against gravity (toe standing and squatting), lateral weight shift, and axial rotation (Fig. 34b,c). Initial patterns of independent standing though, lack rotational components. Instead, infants assume a broad stance with both legs in abduction and external rotation. This is similar to the pattern of the Landau reaction. The first steps take them along the crib in a lateral cruising pattern. The same broad base is maintained when they finally venture to walk independently. The first gait pattern is characterized by lateral flexion of the trunk and a primitive flexor pattern of the advancing leg. Until they apply pelvic rotation when walking, the infants first steps will be very short. Pelvic control is not fully developed in this position and the pronounced extension of the trunk combined with the high guard position of the arms seems to compensate. The infant pulls to standing, moving quickly through a half-kneeling position when unable to maintain balance. Postural alignment and balance gradually become more and more refined (Figs. 35 and 36).

ABNORMAL

Standing and walking are considerably delayed in abnormal development. Without appropriate intervention, the resulting gait pattern reflects most obviously the imbalance between different motor components.

Predominant hypertonicity. Abnormal tonus affects the standing posture considerably and leads to poor postural alignment. Hypertonicity and the exaggerated positive supporting reaction cause plantarflexion, and weight bearing occurs exclusively on the ball of the foot. Flexion, adduction, and internal rotation of hips facilitate pronation of forefoot and eversion of heel. This is a very poor support base and tends to accentuate abnormal developmental patterns throughout the body (Fig. 37). In infants whose pelvis is too far back relative to the base of support, the head and trunk are used to bring forward the center of gravity, thus increasing hip flexion even more (Fig. 38). The infant with strong hypertonicity of the legs cannot half kneel

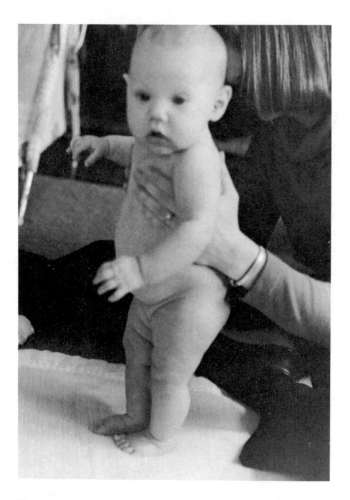

Figure 34a (Normal). During early phases of supported standing, the infant is unable to bring the hips forward for vertical alignment of feet, hips, and shoulders. Weight bearing on the heels occurs with the knees in neutral extension.

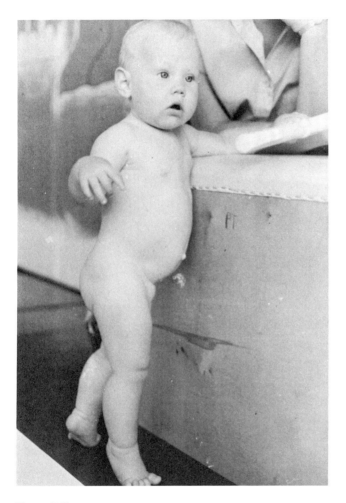

Figure 34b (Normal). While supporting herself, this infant moves between extended and flexed postures (toe standing and squatting). The center of gravity is now brought forward (8 months).

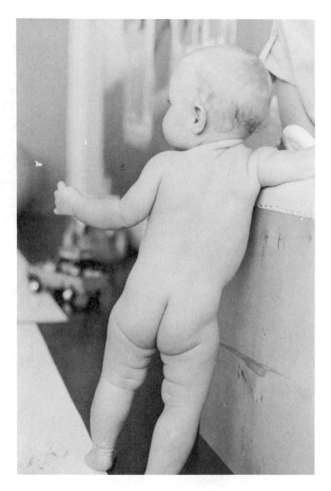

Figure 34c (Normal). Lateral weight shift and axial rotation are further skills which the infant practices in supported standing before attempting to walk (8 to 9 months).

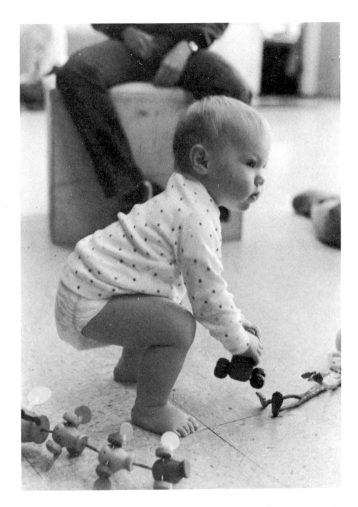

Figure 35 (Normal). A good sense of balance is expressed in the ability to squat without support (12 to 13 months).

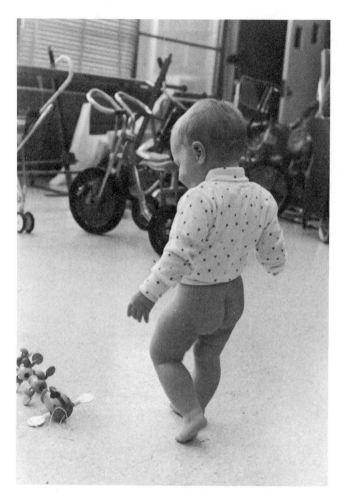

Figure 36 (Normal). After the infant has learned to walk independently, efforts to refine balance and posture must continue. Although this 12-month-old infant no longer demonstrates the "high-guard" posturing of the arms, scapular retraction indicates that rotation within the body axis is not yet fully mastered during walking.

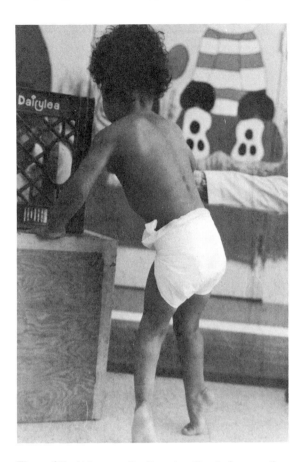

Figure 37 (Abnormal). Toe standing is frequently seen in abnormal development. Postural tonus, alignment, and balance, however, contrast greatly with the adaptations of the normal baby. Compare with Fig. 34b.

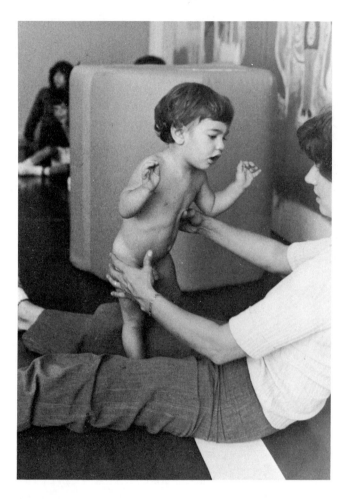

Figure 38 (Abnormal). The center of gravity cannot be aligned over the base of support without pelvic and hip control This results in compensatory patterns of trunk, head and arms. Compare with Fig. 34a. (Photography by Carol Herwig.)

and the great effort exerted to stand up increases the abnormal extensor pattern, causing weight bearing to shift to the dorsum of the feet.

Hypotonicity. The hypotonic infant may initially bear full weight only on the heel while curling the forefoot up in dorsiflexion and clawing the toes. In contrast to the hypertonic pattern, hypotonicity allows for wide abduction and exaggerated external rotation which shifts the weight also to the medial side of the foot and interferes with the development of proper balance reactions. The infant lacks active hip extension and pelvic control which affects postural alignment of trunk and head.

NORMAL AND ABNORMAL FEEDING PATTERNS

The vital behavior of successful feeding is insured from the onset through strong feeding reflexes: the rooting, suck-swallow, bite, and gag reflexes. These are already developed in the fetus and are active in utero. After birth, the different feeding reflexes must be coordinated with one more function: respiration. This coordination also seems to be prepared in utero where rhythmic expansions of the rib cage have been observed in combination with sucking motions [2]. A rhythmic interplay exists between sucking, swallowing, and breathing, determined by the sucking reflex [7]. From the beginning, the normal infant demonstrates some flexibility in this highly reflexive behavior and the capability to adjust to a variety of feeding situations. Infantile feeding reflexes become modified in the growing infant and, gradually, more mature feeding patterns emerge. For a more detailed description of feeding patterns see Chapter 6 (Observation of Feeding Patterns).

CNS impairment frequently causes disturbances of this highly coordinated and complex behavior and abnormal oral development is, thus, often detected at a very early age. When feeding reflexes are weak and difficult to elicit, tube feeding is often initiated. Choking and aspiration may result when coordination between the different feeding reflexes and breathing is disorganized and may be life-threatening. Adaptability of feeding behavior is often poor, which restricts the infant to rigid feeding procedures and limited diets, often resulting in nutritional deficits. As with primitive postural reflexes, primitive and exaggerated feeding reflexes may persist, resulting in stereotyped feeding behavior which interferes with function as the child grows older. Feeding sessions may become unreasonably long, while much food and its nourishment is lost due to uncoordinated and abnormal swallowing patterns.

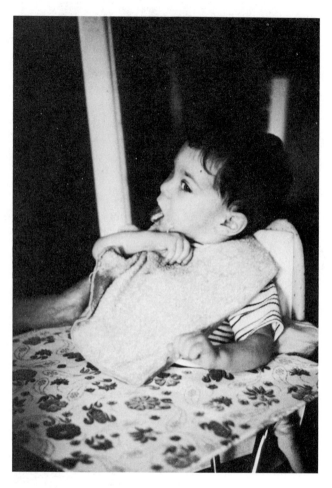

Figure 39 (Abnormal) Jaw and tongue thrusting accompany tonic reflex behavior and are also an expression of exaggerated primitive feeding reflexes. (From *The Infant with Cerebral Palsy: An Approach to Identification, Management, and Treatment*, A. L. Scherzer. Private printing, New York, 1973.)

Facial and oral motor functions cannot be separated from other behavior. Postural functions, such as head control, trunk control, and shoulder girdle posture have a strong effect on oral motor patterns. Without postural stability along the spine, compensatory hypertonicity is likely to occur in oral and pharyngeal areas. Predominant hypertonicity in the oral and facial area impede fine coordinated and dissociated oral movements. Jaw thrusting, tongue thrusting, and retraction of lips and/or tongue accompany dominating tonic reflexes (Fig. 39). Predominant postural asymmetry or ATNR posturing are also reflected in the oral posture and, if combined with abnormal tonus, may lead to subluxation or dislocation of the mandible.

Distorted reactions toward sensory stimuli, such as hypersensitivity to touch and/or temperature, taste, and smell aggravate abnormal tonus. The infant may, as a result, give the appearance of total avoidance, adding even more frustration and tension to an already anxiety-filled and difficult feeding procedure. Positive interactions and communication between mother and infant as it normally emerges during feeding is curtailed. Instead of the enjoyable opportunity for social interaction, mealtimes become burdensome and a struggle for both infant and caregiver.

Hypersensitivity toward sensory stimulation may also interfere with mouthing, thus depriving the infant of an important avenue of learning about properties of objects in preparation for future perceptual and cognitive development. Refinement of feeding skills, as it occurs during normal development also serves as preparation for other nonfeeding functions, such as articulation and speech. Primitive and abnormal feeding patterns delay or prevent normal sound and speech production. Abnormal swallowing patterns and abnormal posture of jaws, lips, and tongue result in excessive drooling. Abnormal oral function may impair dental health and contributes significantly to the development of oral and facial deformities, such as malocclusions and deformities of the palate.

REFERENCES

1. Hooker, D. The Prenatal Origin of Behavior. New York, Hafner, 1969.

2. Milani-Comparetti, A., Janniruberto, A., Tajani, E. Fetal Movements and Cerebral Palsy. Proceedings from Development of Movement in Infancy, pp. 1-37. Division of Physical Therapy, University of North Carolina, Chapel Hill, 1981.

3. Bly, L. The Components of Normal and Abnormal Movements During the First Year of Life. Proceedings from Development of Movment in Infants, pp. 85-135. Division of Physical Therapy, University of North Carolina, Chapel Hill, N.C., 1981.

4. Bobath, B., and Bobath, K. Motor Development in the Different Types of Cerebral Palsy. London, Heinemann, 1975.

5. Quinton, M. B. Normal and Abnormal Development. Course in Neuro-developmental Treatment. Unpublished lecture notes, Seattle, Washington, 1978.

6. Quinton, M. B. Normal and Abnormal Development During the First Year of Life. NDT Baby Course. Unpublished lecture notes, Roosevelt, New York, 1981.

7. Peiper, A. Cerebral Function in Infancy and Childhood, New York, Consultants Bureau, 1963.

BIBLIOGRAPHY

André-Thomas, and Autgaerden, S. Locomotion From Pre- to Post-Natal Life. Clinics in Developmental Medicine, No. 24. London, The Spastics Society Medical Education and Information Unit in associated with Heinemann, 1966.

Bèbe, M. Mi Hijo Su Primer Ano. Buenos Aires, Sigmar, 1979.

Blankenstein, M. van., Welbergen, U. R., and Haas, J. H. de. Le Développment Du Nourrisson. Paris, Presses Universitaires, 1962.

Bobath, B., and Bobath, K. Motor Development In The Different Types of Cerebral Palsy. London, Heinemann, 1975.

Bower, T. G. R. Development in Infancy. San Francisco, Freeman, 1974.

Brazelton, T. B. Infants and Mothers, Differences in Development, New York, Dell, 1969.

Brazelton, T. B. Toddlers and Parents, a Declaration of Independence. New York, Delacorte, 1974.

Caplan, F. (Ed.). The First Twelve Months of Life, Your Baby's Growth Month by Month. New York, Grosset & Dunlap, 1973.

Caplan, F., and Caplan, T. The Second Twelve Months of Life, a Kaleidoscope of Growth. New York, Grosset & Dunlap, 1979.

Casaer, P. Postural Behavior in Newborn Infants. Philadelphia, Lippincott, 1979.

Gesell, A., and Amatruda, C. S. Developmental Diagnosis: Normal and Abnormal Child Development. New York, Hoeber, 1947.

Illingworth, R. S. The Development of the Infant and Young Child, Normal and Abnormal (3rd ed.). London, Livingstone, 1967.

Milani-Comparetti, A., and Gidoni, E. A. Pattern analysis of motor development and its disorders. *Dev. Med. Child. Neurol.* 9:626-630, 1967.

Prechtl, H. Continuity of Neural Functions from Prenatal to Postnatal Life. Clinics in Developmental Medicine No. 94. London, Heinemann, 1985.

Saint-Anne Dargassies, S. Neurological Development in the Full-Term and Premature Neonate. Amsterdam, Elsevier, 1977.

Stern, F. The reflex development of the infant. *Am. J. Occup. Ther.* 25: 155-158, 1971.

Touwen, B. Neurological Development in Infancy. Clinics in Developmental Medicine No. 58. London, Heinemann, 1976.

White, B. The First Three Years of Life. Englewood Cliffs, NJ, Prentice-Hall, 1975.

5

Neurodevelopmental Assessment of Infants: Concepts

OVERVIEW

Symptoms resulting from damage to the maturing central nervous system (CNS) vary considerably between individual patients. The picture presented by each patient also changes drastically during the course of development. The wide scope of abnormal development has been compared with the normal baby in Chapter 4. The assessment of cerebral palsy and related sensorimotor deficits cannot follow a routine approach, but must be adapted to the individual patient. However, the underlying general concepts remain uniform for all patients.

A general orientation to assessment of infants is presented. Sensorimotor and adaptive behavior are analyzed from various points of reference. This allows grouping of the vast variety of reactions into few categories. In each category normal and abnormal behavior are contrasted with each other.

GENERAL ORIENTATION

Holistic Approach

The major focus of the therapist's assessment is the analysis of postural reactions and motor skills, including feeding. Postural evaluation must, however, go beyond the testing for various postural reflexes in an artificial testing situation. The therapist should instead observe how different postural reactions are coordinated with each other, how they are used spontaneously, and how they are adapted to different situations. Motor development cannot be separated from social, communicative, and intellectual skills. Furthermore, the evaluation process must be expanded to the infant/parent (family) unit. Sensory experiences and possible sensory restrictions must be considered.

Patterns of Posture and Movement

The major problem of the patient with cerebral palsy is not caused by a dysfunction of individual muscles or muscle groups, but by a lack of coordination of muscle action. This is expressed in characteristic patterns of posture and movement, as well as in an imbalance between different motor patterns. The motor repertoire is restricted to few and stereotyped patterns while mature postural reactions are impaired. Persistence of primitive and poorly integrated motor patterns necessitates more and more abnormal compensations as the motor tasks the infant attempts become more difficult. During early phases of development these abnormal motor patterns may alternate with more normal patterns. Identification of abnormal development based on disturbed patterns of posture and movements was introduced by Dr. Karel and Berta Bobath as a major concept of the neurodevelopmental treatment (NDT) approach.

Quality of Motor Patterns

Mere achievement of early developmental milestones is not a reliable sign of normal development. Rather, the quality of sensorimotor behavior relative to accompanying postures and intrinsic movement components must be considered.

Automatic Postural Reactions

Functional activities, developmental motor skills and volitional motor acts are performed on the basis of automatic postural reactions, such as the organization of postural tonus and of reciprocal innervation, righting and equilibrium reactions. Development of these motor patterns is crucial for the development of antigravity posture and efficient, controlled movement patterns. The interplay between different righting reactions provides a change of position and a means of progression, such as rolling, creeping, etc. Equilibrium reactions provide postural control and balance.

ADAPTIVE BEHAVIOR

Immaturity and dysfunction of the central nervous system are frequently expressed in general attitudes and responsiveness to environmental stimuli. The quality of certain adaptive responses can therefore strengthen or weaken the significance of suspect abnormal motor signs, specifically during early phases of development.

Threshold for Stimulation

CNS dysfunction can be detected in the infant's intolerance to different stimuli. During the first weeks of life, normal babies display an ability to adapt to a variety of stimuli and to organize themselves accordingly. They can adjust to disturbing stimuli and, to some extent, protect themselves against overstimulation. Once aroused, infants find various ways of calming themselves.

The infant with CNS dysfunction may demonstrate an abnormally low threshold to stimulation. This hypersensitivity can produce highly disorganized behavior and irritability. Hypersensitivity may be revealed in the infant's reaction to auditory and visual stimuli and to being touched. Conversely, the extremely "good" infant may be exhibiting a lack of responsiveness and abnormally high threshold to stimulation due to CNS impairment.

Variability of Behavior

Infants learn very early to modify their responses as well as to adapt to new situations. Variability and unpredictability of responses, including patterns of primitive reflexes, are important characteristics in normal development.

A very narrow repertoire of responses, and stereotyped behavior in areas of sensorimotor, social, emotional, and mental functions, indicate abnormality.

Mental Responsiveness

Alertness and attentiveness are exhibited by the newborn, although only for short periods at a time. The skill for selective attention to environmental stimuli starts to develop early and is very important for further mental development.

A lack of initiative and respondence may occur with abnormal development. Pronounced distractability is another expression of CNS immaturity; it reduces the opportunity for early learning and may aggrevate developmental delay. Untiring repetition of stereotyped responses to the same stimulus contrasts equally with the typical response of normal babies. They quickly tire of too much repetition and seem to strive for a constant expansion into new experiences.

Social Interaction

Interest in their surroundings, curiosity, and clearly displayed pleasure in communication are characteristic of the healthy and normally developing infant. Babies make extreme efforts to achieve personal attention and seem to thrive on it.

Social interaction and responses to the environment may be suppressed and disturbed in infants with CNS impairment.

MOTOR SKILLS AND DEVELOPMENTAL MILESTONES

Motor output cannot be separated from sensory input. Movements are shaped by proprioceptive and tactile feedback and by visual, auditory, and labyrinthine orientation. A motor act is often prompted by visual or auditory stimuli. Quality and type of sensory experiences provided by the infant's environment must be considered as much as any sensory deficit.

A list of functional skills achieved by the infant as well as age-appropriate skills not obtained form one part of the assessment. Allocation of the infant's level of functioning to specific months and weeks, however, cannot reflect the true developmental deficiencies but can misrepresent the infant's true condition, especially when achievement of developmental skills is scattered.

The following outline organizes functional skills into major categories. The developmental level within each category must be adjusted to the child's chronological age and developmental stage. This section describes *what* the infant can do, independently or with assistance, efficiently or with effort.

Positional Control and Balance

The ability to balance and function in any or all of the following positions is assessed according to age and impairment: prone, supine, sidelying; quadruped, standing. Which of these positions is most/least functional and which position is most often used by the infant? The nonambulatory infant is placed into supported standing to evaluate the capability for weight bearing through the legs. The parachute reaction may be evaluated in vertical suspension: It consists of a protective reaction of the legs during sudden displacement of the erect trunk and it emerges at 4 months (Milani-Comparetti).

The legs assume a posture of extension and abduction while the feet dorsiflex.

Upper Extremity Function

The skill in propping on arms or hands is observed in prone and in sitting. A test for protective extension of the arms in all directions is included when appropriate.

Hand functions, such as reach, grasp, and release are evaluated for voluntary control. Bilateral manipulation as well as the ability to transfer objects are skills to look for. A strong preference for one hand is suggestive of sensory or tonal asymmetries. Consistent fisting of the hands is abnormal. Hand play, body investigation, and mouthing are important stages of normal motor development.

Change of Positions

The ability to change positions is a significant motor function. Rolling from prone to supine and vice versa, moving from prone to crawling position, assuming a sitting position, and pulling to standing all give the infant some measure of independence. Some infants may require assistance to be successful in their attempts.

Progression

Ability for and mode of progression are described next. A baby can move around by rolling, belly crawling, crawling on hands and knees or hands and feet, cruising, or walking. Some infants learn to progress in sitting; for example, the infant with hemiplegia who propels forward with one hand while 'dragging' the hemiplegic side along; the same retraction of the hemiplegic side may also be seen in walking. When assessing gait, the therapist prompts the child to walk in all directions, turn, and stand up with or without support. When asked to ascend or descend stairs, many infants regress to crawling.

Activities of Daily Living (ADL)

How the infant is being carried and dressed is assessed according to the infant's adaptation to caregiving and also to the parents' adapting to the infant's disability. How does the sensory cueing that the infant receives relate to the motor responses observed? Bathing is another important caregiving activity to be observed during a home visit.

Oromotor Function

This includes mouthing, feeding, and positional control of jaw and mouth at rest and during movement.

Communication

Interaction between parent and infant may give important cues on how to approach the infant. Does the baby initiate interaction, play with sounds, use words, understand speech? Any suspect hearing deficits need further follow-up.

QUALITY OF MOTOR PATTERNS

Abnormal development is most obvious when age—appropriate motor skills are lacking and when developmental milestones are not reached. Early identification however, requires a more qualitative assessment including quality of postural tonus and of motor patterns. During the course of development, patterns of previously acquired skills are more and more refined, postural mechanisms become more complex, more sophisticated, and, more efficient. Quality of movement patterns reflects the level of maturation and integrative function of the CNS. Well-integrated sensorimotor behavior precedes development of numerous perceptual and cognitive skills. The quality of movements has, therefore, farreaching impact on the child's future. While the previous section describes function or what the infant can do, this section describes *how* it is done.

Knowledge of normal motor patterns and how they change in the course of development is an important tool for early identification of abnormal sensorimotor behavior. The most important normal and abnormal motor patterns are described in Chapter 4.

Postural Tonus

Postural tonus reflects the dynamic interplay between excitatory and inhibitory centers of the CNS and is receptive to exteroceptive, proprioceptive, and interoceptive stimuli. Consequently, degree and distribution of postural tonus are changeable and can be influenced by the type and quality of sensory input.

NORMAL

Strength and Distribution. Quality and distribution of postural tonus are expressed in patterns of posture and movements, and in the degree of ease or effort during movements. Normal postural tonus is sufficiently high to enable weight bearing and support against gravity. Yet at the same time normal postural tonus is low enough to allow quick and easy adaptations toward active and passive movements.

Distribution of tonus changes during the course of development. During early phases, tonus is higher distally than proximally (Saint-Anne Dargassies, 1977). This pattern is completely reversed providing relatively more proximal stability and more distal motility.*

Reciprocal Innervation. Stability, motility, and the interplay between both is determined by reciprocal innervation which coordinates opposing muscle groups. With normal motor control a movement initiated by one muscle group (agonist) is guided by the gradual relaxation and elongation of the opposing muscle group (antagonist). When agonist and antagonist work with the same force, cocontraction occurs, resulting in postural stabilization.*

ABNORMAL

CNS deficit causes an imbalance between centers of excitation and inhibition. Distribution of tonus differs from the norm and may reflect patterns of abnormal tonic reflex behavior. When distribution of tonus fails to undergo normal developmental changes, tonus remains high distally while it is low proximally. Balancing and manipulative skills are then impeded.

Poor support tonus, lack of righting against gravity, and restrictions of mobility may be expressed in the patient's spontaneous motor behavior. A more precise, qualitative assessment of tonus is achieved when the therapist handles the infant. Abnormal postural tonus is indicated in the child's inability to adapt to the therapist's handling.

Postural tonus may change drastically, depending on the infant's position, activity, state of excitement, and amount of effort used. Therefore, tonus mut be evaluated during different activities and in different situations, that is, when the infant is at rest as well as when active and exposed to different stimuli.

Hypertonicity and Spasticity. In the case of hypertonicity, the examiner feels undue resistance toward antigravity movements and undue assistance

---

*For more information on the Postural Reflex Mechanism please see Chapter 9.

when moving with gravity. The degree of resistance may fluctuate throughout the range of a given movement. Strong resistance may suddenly disappear at a certain point (clasp knife phenomenon). Hypertonicity is also evidenced in associated reactions, for example, during commando crawling where the infant pulls forward with the arms which increases extensor hypertonicity of the legs. Clonus is another phenomenon associated with spasticity.

Hypotonicity. The hypotonic infant also lacks proper postural control against gravity. The limbs and body sink into gravity which is expressed for example, in the typical posture of the limbs often referred to as "frog position." When moved passively, the limbs feel heavy because the infant cannot support their weight. Lacking resistance toward extreme movements, hypotonic infants often display hypermobility. Hypertonicity often can be provoked in the basically hypotonic infant with stress and brisk handling, for example, in a test for adductor hypertonicity.

Fluctuations of Tonus and Tremor. Strong fluctuations of tonus can be felt in patients with athetosis. Involuntary movements, so typical for the athetoid patient, may be, to some degree, the result of these fluctuations. Tremor can often be observed in the ataxic child.

Disturbed Reciprocal Innervation. Disturbances of interplay between agonist and antagonist vary. The spastic patient applies too much cocontraction, that is, agonist and antagonist work with the same force. As a result, movements are restricted and require much effort. In the athetoid patient, a paucity of sustained cocontraction contributes to a lack of postural stabilization, leading to uncontrolled and exaggerated movements.

Variability of Motor Responses

NORMAL
From the onset, normal babies demonstrate a certain variability in motor responses even in their reflex behavior. During the course of development, certain motor patterns may dominate but different or opposing motor patterns are not totally excluded. For example, by 6 months of age, the baby seems to practice predominantly patterns of extension, especially when prone. When supine, however, the same baby plays frequently with patterns of flexion, i.e., raising legs, reaching toward knees and feet.

ABNORMAL
Stereotyped movements and predominant motor patterns displayed more or less exclusively in various positions indicate central nervous system (CNS) dysfunction.

Grading of Movements

NORMAL

Grading of movements for amplitude, speed, and velocity requires integration between diverse sensory feedback systems with control centers for motor output. Motor responses must be adapted according to labyrinthine, visual, proprioceptive, tactile, and auditory feedback. Grading of movements in space is prepared through grading of movements during weight bearing and weight shifting.

ABNORMAL

In the abnormally developing child, this learning process may be interrupted by the sensory feedback and/or motor control systems. Visual and auditory feedback, for example, are inaccurate and poorly integrated when the infant has poor head control. Abnormal postural alignment of the head also influences the labyrinthine feedback. Poor postural stability, such as lack of trunk control and poor proximal stabilization of the shoulder girdle interferes with graded reaching among other motor functions. Movements are jerky and the infant overshoots when reaching. Some infants achieve outside stability for grasping or releasing objects by leaning on arm and hand. Abnormal postural tonus also prevents the execution of graded and smooth movements. Fluctuations of tonus, involuntary movements, and tremor which may be evident at a later stage of development, make it very difficult to develop well-coordinated and efficient movement patterns. Paucity of movements or excessive, disorganized movements are further symptoms of possible CNS impairment. Sensory deficits also delay or alter motor development.

Sequencing of Movements

NORMAL

Each righting reaction is facilitatory to and may elicit other righting as well as equilibrium reactions resulting in a chain reaction or sequencing of movement patterns. Lateral head righting, for example, results in lateral righting of the trunk which, in turn, causes the limbs to assume a posture of the amphibian reaction or a balance response. The sequential activation of righting and equilibrium reactions engulfs the whole body and provides the infant with such important motor functions as change of position in space or progression.

ABNORMAL

Sequencing of movements is hampered when the development of righting and equilibrium reactions is delayed or disturbed. A smooth sequential flow of movements is often blocked by the predominance of one motor pattern or by the excessive use of one part of the body, for example, by the infant who uses arms and upper trunk as compensation for lack of motor control in legs and pelvis. A wide base of support, such as the "frog position" of the limbs or the "W sitting" position, poses a mechanical obstacle to changes of posture and disturbs the sequencing of movements. These infants then present a quite static picture which contrasts sharply with the dynamic motor behavior of a normal baby.

Integration of Primitive Reflexes

The primitive reflexes which are most often described by clinicians are the Moro reflex and the tonic reflexes, that is, the tonic labyrinthine reflex (TLR), the asymmetrical tonic neck reflex (ATNR), and the symmetrical tonic neck reflex (STNR). A reliable prognostic relation between a classic reflex test and functional motor skills is now widely questioned.

NORMAL
These reflexes are present at birth or appear during the first weeks of life. Infants with normal CNS development can make easy progress from these primitive reflex patterns because more purposeful actions can override them. With the maturation of the CNS these primitive reflexes are modified and integrated into more complex postural reactions and are then no longer displayed in their pure form.

ABNORMAL
In infants whose CNS development is impaired, the primitive reflexes are not adaptable, and may be exaggerated and stereotyped, although the classical tonic reflexes are rarely seen in their pure form. Deficient maturation of postural mechanisms results in such infants adhering to these primitive motor patterns. When used to excess, the patterns become ever more inefficient for achieving more complex actions. The undue effort leads to increased hypertonicity, which in turn, makes the postural adaptations even more dysfunctional.

Postural Symmetry

NORMAL
The development of symmetry and midline orientation is extremely important and a prerequisite for many perceptual skills. Integration between the two sides must take place before a higher form of laterality and reciprocality

and, finally, dominance of one side can develop (three years). During the first year of life, predominant patterns of postural symmetry and asymmetry alternate repeatedly at an ever higher level of control and dissociation.

ABNORMAL

Highly associated patterns of asymmetry often predominate. The lack of midline orientation and bilateral hand activities may lead to distortion of body image and body awareness and may severely hamper the ability to learn about properties of different objects. Primitive symmetrical patterns interfere with the development of laterality and reciprocality.

Postural Alignment

With the influence of righting reactions, infants learn to right themselves against gravity, assuming a normal position of the head in space and maintaining or restoring proper postural alignment between head, trunk, and limbs. In each body plane there are different motor patterns associated with righting reactions.

Plane 1. Righting in the Sagittal Plane (Extension and Flexion Against Gravity)

NORMAL

Although the development of postural control starts with patterns of extension against gravity, more mature patterns of righting in the sagittal plane require coordination between axial extension and flexion and the ability for caudal weight shifting to allow head, arms, and trunk to move freely against gravity. Development of postural control is in a cephalo to caudal direction. Once stability through the spine is established, the limbs can be moved against gravity, as in the Landau reaction, that is, in ventral suspension the whole body extends against gravity with the hips in extension, abduction, external rotation, and with the feet dorsiflexed. Gradually, differentiated movements of the limbs, such as forward reach with extended elbows, or lifting of extended legs while supine become possible.

ABNORMAL

Postural tonus. Instead of righting against gravity, the infant may sink into gravity (hypotonicity) or be pulled into gravity (hypertonicity). Progravity pull is especially strong when tonic reflexes dominate motor behavior. Hypertonicity increases the more the infant tries to move against gravity. Effort and stress have the same effect.

Coordination Between Flexion and Extension. The fine interplay between extension and flexion is often disturbed in the presence of CNS impairment. While these infants may be able to move against gravity to some extent, postural alignment is abnormal and motor components are poorly integrated (see Chap. 4).

Dominant Extensor Patterns. When patterns of extension predominate, the cervical and lumbar spine are pulled into excessive lordosis. The head retracts while the chin juts forward. The neck cannot elongate without the development of flexion against gravity. Without the counterbalance of flexion the pelvis is pulled into an anterior tilt which interferes with the development of full hip extension. Further development of righting and balancing in all body planes is severely hampered.

Compensatory Flexion. Predominant flexion frequently occurs as a compensatory pattern, especially in more upright positions such as sitting or during crawling. The abnormal pull into flexion is then superimposed on early (extensor) patterns developed in prone and supine.

Plane 2. Righting in the Frontal Plane (Lateral Flexion)

NORMAL
Proper postural alignment in the frontal plane requires lateral righting: a pattern of side flexion of neck and trunk toward the non-weight-bearing side together with active elongation and extension on the weight-bearing side. With progressive lateral displacement, axial rotation becomes more obvious. Lateral righting is only possible when total patterns of extension and flexion are inhibited and, therefore, seems to be a significant milestone in the course of development.

ABNORMAL
Lateral righting is not developed when total and synergic patterns of extension and flexion prevail. Although lateral trunk flexion is often substituted for trunk rotation, a close observation of the postural alignment reveals considerable differences in the quality and efficiency of the response when compared with a true righting response. In abnormal development, lateral flexion does not provide a good postural alignment since it is often combined with predominant extension of the spine. Shoulder girdle and pelvic girdle are not aligned in the frontal plane. There is no active elongation on the weight-bearing side. However, mechanical stability can be achieved in the end range of vertebral joints.

Plane 3. Righting in the Transverse Plane (Rotation Within the Body Axis)

NORMAL

Rotation within the body axis develops with the influence of body righting on the body. It is an essential component of a wide variety of functional skills such as change of position (for example, sidelying to sitting, sitting to crawling). In addition, righting within the body axis can be observed in segmental rolling. Between prone and supine, rolling is initiated from the pelvis; between supine and prone, rolling is initiated from head and shoulders. In more upright positions, such as sitting, the development of rotation allows trunk control and frees the arms for manipulation of toys and refinement of hand function. Rotation can be combined with a weight shift to the opposite side as in equilibrium reactions or to the same side as in the transition between sitting and quadruped.

ABNORMAL

Patients with CNS deficit frequently fail to develop rotation within the body axis and the resulting refined form of balancing. Side flexion of the head and trunk is often substituted and balancing requires undue effort. The infant has to rely on a broad base of support, namely wide abduction of the limbs, which encourages static positions. Furthermore, the arms must be used for protection against falling because of poor trunk control. Play activities and manipulation of objects are consequently restricted.

Postural Stability and Motility

Every movement displaces the center of gravity and requires postural adjustments which increase in complexity with a decrease of outside support. Controlled movement requires a counterbalance of postural stability. This postural stability must be adjusted at every phase of the movements. Efficient postural stability is, therefore, dynamic. Controlled movements of the extremities are based on proximal stability. Controlled movements of the body in space are made possible through the development of equilibrium reactions.

Dynamic Proximal Stability

NORMAL

In accordance with the cephalo to caudal and proximal to distal sequence of development, postural stability is first seen in the upper trunk and shoulder girdle, and later in the pelvic girdle. Postural stability is developed through weight bearing. The infant can perform fine controlled movements of the upper extremities in space only after achieving dynamic stability of the shoulder girdle and trunk through activities of weight bearing and weight shifting of the upper extremities (by about 5 to 6 months of age). Controlled and isolated finger movements require, in addition, good stability of elbow and wrist. Efficient head and trunk control is made possible through the development of weight shifting through lower trunk and pelvis. Balancing activities of the lower extremities and feet require postural control of trunk and pelvis.

ABNORMAL

Lack of proximal stability causes difficulties in midline control for all body planes: proper alignment between head, shoulder, and pelvic girdle cannot be achieved. Weight shifting is often occasioned by movements of the head (head tilting toward weight-bearing side or into gravity), which directly opposes proper righting, and balance reactions (head and trunk tilting against gravity). Further development of head and trunk control is consequently hampered and manipulative skills are not fully developed. Motor patterns of the lower extremities become increasingly abnormal.

Patterns of Fixation. The infant who lacks proper patterns of weight shifting, righting, and balancing tries to obtain some postural stability with abnormal patterns of fixation. In contrast with normal postural stability, these patterns of fixation are static and interfere with efficient weight shifting; and in time, lead to contractures. They occur most often around shoulder and pelvic girdle and are expressed, for example, in elevation of shoulders or anterior pelvic tilt. A broad base of support (i.e., wide abduction of the limbs) may also be used for postural stability resulting again in a static posture. Another form of abnormal postural fixation occurs at distal points of the limbs, especially in the hypotonic infant who tends to stabilize by leaning on the lateral and ulnar side of hands and feet. A distal point of fixation is also achieved by crossing the feet which is often seen when the infant sits.

Equilibrium Reactions

NORMAL

While righting reactions provide postural alignment, equilibrium reactions maintain and restore balance through tonal adjustments or compensatory movements. Equilibrium reactions build on and modify righting reactions. They appear at the age of about 6 months and emerge first in prone, then in supine, then in sitting, in quadruped, and, finally, in standing and walking. By the time a full repertoire of equilibrium reactions is achieved, the child is 5 to 6 years old. It is interesting to note that the infant is already sitting unsupported when first equilibrium reactions in prone position develop. The same temporal overlapping of motor functions occurs between sitting and standing and standing and walking. Balance reactions in standing and walking emerge during the second year of life and include, in addition to proximal postural adjustments, compensatory steps in all directions as well as intrinsic, compensatory movements of forefoot and toes. In subsequent years, postural adjustments become more refined. Patterns of equilibrium reactions depend on the direction of displacement, which is mostly asymmetrical and elicits a pattern of axial rotation of head and trunk and a "reaching pattern" of the extremities. The pattern of the extremities depends on the direction of the weight shift; usually it incorporates some degree of external rotation and extension.

The subtle and quick postural adjustments of the equilibrium reactions can only occur when a high degree of differentiation of movement patterns is achieved. (For more information on the Postural Reflex Mechanism please see Chap. 9.)

ABNORMAL
Primitive and total movement patterns, limitations as to mobility, and abnormal postural tonus interfere with the performance of equilibrium reactions.

Protective Extension of the Arms

NORMAL
Protective extension of the arms is applied when other balance reactions are insufficient. Its development precedes and partially overlaps with that of other equilibrium reactions. By about 5 to 6 months, the infant leans on slightly fisted hands when sitting unsupported. During the following weeks, greater wrist mobility develops, allowing better extension of wrist and fingers with stronger extension throughout the arm. Protective extension of the arms forward, sideways, and backward develops between 6 and 12 months of age.

ABNORMAL
The infant who lacks dynamic shoulder girdle and trunk stability cannot develop efficient patterns of upper extremity weight bearing. Also, protective extension of the arms is normally combined with appropriate head righting. Any delay or disturbance in the development of righting reactions interferes with the development of appropriate protective extension of the arms.

Dissociation of Movements (Mature Versus Primitive Motor Patterns)

NORMAL

The ability to combine components of different patterns, such as patterns of flexion and extension, requires an inhibitory control and develops, therefore, only gradually with progressive CNS maturation. Total motor patterns must be inhibited for isolated and differentiated movements to occur. Dissociation of total motor patterns allows formation of a vast variety of new movement patterns and provides the postural mechanism for all skillful motor activities.

A very primitive and preparatory function of dissociation may be seen in the ATNR posture, where each side of the body assumes a different pattern. Righting reactions and the amphibian reaction evolve with further development of inhibitory control and suppress the ATNR. Some other patterns of dissociation have been described in Chapter 4.

Differentiation of proximal movements precedes those occurring distally. Progression is cephalo to caudal; therefore, dissociation between movements of head, shoulder girdle, and trunk—as seen for example, during lateral weight shifting in prone on elbows or hands—occurs before the infant is able to dissociate pelvic movements from movements of the trunk. Such dissociation enables the infant, for example, to rotate the pelvis back during rolling or when prone so as to sit. Dissociation between movements of leg and pelvis express an even later stage of development and changes, for example, the gait pattern eliminating the pronounced lateral hiking of the pelvis while the hip flexes during the swing phase. The pattern of heel strike as seen in the mature gait pattern indicates differentiation of movement patterns throughout the whole body. As with the development of rotation, these skills must be conquered in each position. For instance, dissociation of movements of hip, knee, and ankle is applied in prone, then while sitting and crawling before it can be incorporated into the mature gait pattern.

ABNORMAL

The development of dissociation and differentiation of movement patterns is disturbed in combination with sensorimotor deficits. Primitive and synergic motor patterns persist and become increasingly inefficient for higher and complex motor tasks. Compensatory and abnormal motor patterns emerge, especially when the infant assumes more upright positions, and the gap between normal and abnormal motor behavior widens.

PRIMARY ABNORMAL PATTERNS AND COMPENSATORY ABNORMAL PATTERNS

Differentiation between primary abnormal patterns and abnormal patterns that compensate for them is important in designing the treatment program. An approach concerned only with patterns of compensation may reinforce and increase the original abnormality, which in turn, increases the necessity for patterns of compensation; for example, emphasizing extension in the infant who uses compensatory flexion in order to overcome abnormal extension may only elicit more compensatory flexion.

As in normal development, the course of abnormal development also follows a basically cephalo to caudal progression. Primary and initial signs of abnormality, therefore, often include a disturbance of head righting and shoulder girdle and trunk alignment. Also, as in normal development, patterns of extension emerge first and seem to dominate the motor behavior for a prolonged time. Quality and distribution of extension, however, differ from that seen in normal development (see Chap. 4).

Compensatory patterns emerge mostly in more upright positions and with attempts at locomotion. The earliest and most frequently seen is abnormal flexion of upper trunk and neck combined with shoulder elevation and scapular protraction. Flexor hypertonicity may then be superimposed on abnormal extensor tonus.

CONTRACTURES AND DEFORMITIES

An infant who is restricted to few patterns of posture and movement is likely to display limited mobility and may develop contractures and even deformities. A test for mobility is applicable, based on the suspected effects of predominant patterns of posture and movements. To distinguish between movement restrictions due to hypertonicity and the presence of true contractures the infant must be tested while well-aligned and well-supported.

Some of the most obvious factors for the development of contractures and deformities are dominating tonic reflexes (Figs. 1a,1b).

Extensor hypertonicity eventually causes shortening of hip extensors (Fig. 2). Retraction of the shoulders leads to a fixation between the scapula and humerus and, eventually, a winging of the scapula whenever the arm is raised (Fig. 3).

Predominant extensor tonus and a habitual pattern of neck retraction interfere with flexion and elongation of the cervical spine, even in very young infants. Restricted mobility occurs also in other areas of the spine and effects movements of trunk and pelvis.

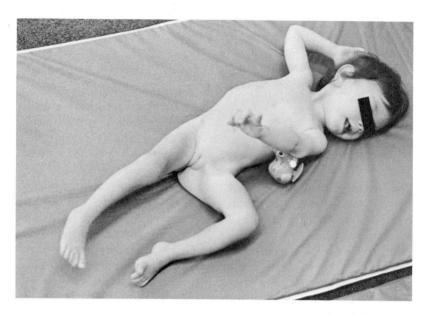

Figure 1a A hypertonic pattern of adduction and internal rotation of the right hip, plantarflexion, and inversion of the right foot is elicited and constantly reinforced by the dominating influence of the ATNR toward the left and may lead to subluxation or dislocation of the right hip.

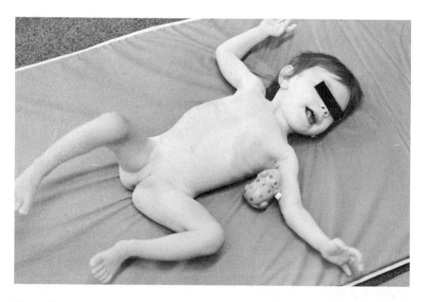

Figure 1b Restricted hip mobility is also demonstrated when the hips are flexed.

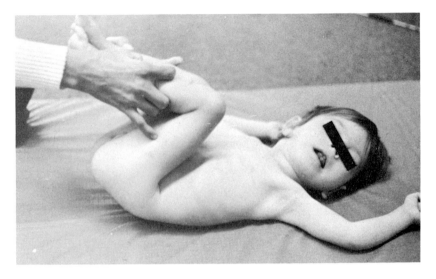

Figure 2 When the legs are elevated beyond 90°, the pelvis is pulled off the support, indicating shortened hip extensors.

Although the hypotonic child tends to display hypermobility in most joints, some contractures may develop due to habitual posturing. For example, a persistent pattern of flexion and abduction of the legs, so typical for the hypotonic patient, may interfere with full hip extension and adduction and may pose problems when the child attempts to stand or walk.

The STNR-posture, which is used by many patients extensively for sitting ("W sitting") and for crawling, soon results in flexor contractures of the legs and may seriously interfere with the development of independent standing and walking.

These are only a few examples. A variety of compensatory patterns emerge, especially in more upright positions and with attempts at locomotion: their impact must be evaluated on an individual basis.

Abnormal patterns of posture and movement as well as abnormal postural tonus can cause severe deformities. Dislocations and subluxations, as mentioned above, are certainly not restricted to the hip joint. In addition to scoliosis, other deformities of the ribcage occur, especially in the infant who does not assume antigravity positions and therefore develops a rather flat and broad rib cage. These deformities can have a severe impact on patterns of respiration and phonation.

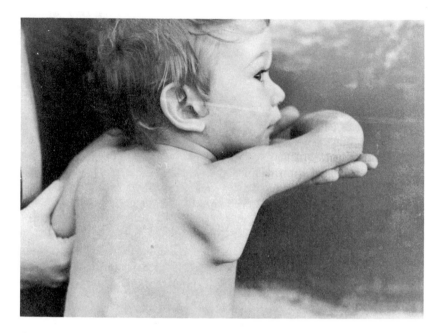

Figure 3 When trunk stability is lacking UE posturing is used in compensation. In time, muscles between scapula and humerus become progressively shorter leading to excessive winging of the scapula whenever the arm is raised (compare with Fig. 34c, Chap. 4).

In order to recommend appropriate methods of prevention, the therapy evaluation must aim to uncover abnormal motor behavior that may be enforcing the development of contractures and deformities.

BIBLIOGRAPHY

André-Thomas, and Autgaerden, S. Locomotion from Pre- to Post-Natal Life. Clinics in Developmental Medicine, No. 24. London, The Spastics Society Medical Education and Information Unit in association with Heinemann, 1966.

André-Thomas, Chesni, I., and Saint-Anne Dargassies, S. The Neurological Examination of the Infant. Clinics in Developmental Medicine, No. 1, London, The Spastic Society Medical Education and Information Unit in association with Heinemann, 1960.

Bèbe, M. Mi Hijo Su Primer Año. Buenos Aires, Sigmar, 1979.

Blankenstein, M. V., Welbergen, U. R., and Haas, J. H. de. Le Développment Du Nourisson. Paris, Presses Universitaires de France, 1962.

Bly, L. The Components of Normal and Abnormal Movement During the First Year of Life. Proceedings from Development of Movement in Infants, May 1980. Division of Physical Therapy, University of North Carolina, Chapel Hill, N.C., 1981.

Bobath, B. Abnormal Postural Reflex Activity Caused by Brain Lesions. (2nd ed.). London, Heinemann, 1971.

Bobath, B., and Bobath, K. Motor Development in the Different Types of Cerebral Palsy. London, Heinemann, 1975.

Bobath, K. The Motor Deficit in Patients with Cerebral Palsy. Clinics in Developmental Medicine, No. 23. London, Heinemann, 1966.

Boehme, R. Improving Upper Body Control. An Approach to Assessment and Treatment of Tonal Dysfunction. Therapy Skill Builders. Tucson, AZ, 1988.

Bosma, J. Form and function in the infant's mouth and pharynx. In Third Symposium on Oral Sensation and Perception. Bosma, J. (Ed.). Springfield, Charles C Thomas, 1972, pp. 3–29.

Bower, T. G. R. Development in Infancy. San Francisco, Freeman, 1974.

Brazelton, T. B. Infants and Mothers, Differences in Development. New York, Dell, 1969.

Brazelton, T. B. Neonatal Behavioral Assessment Scale. Clinics in Developmental Medicine, No. 50. London, The Spastics Society Medical Education and Information Unit in association with Heinemann, 1973.

Brazelton, T. B. Toddlers and Parents, a Declaration of Independence. New York, Delacorte Press, 1974.

Campbell, S. Movement assessment of infants: an evaluation. *Phys. Occ. Ther. Pediatr.* 1(4):53-57, 1981.

Caplan, F. (gen. ed.). The First Twelve Months of Life, Your Baby's Growth Month by Month, New York, Grosset & Dunlap, 1973.

Caplan, F., and Caplan, T. The Second Twelve Months of Life, A Kaleido-scope of Growth. New York, Grosset & Dunlap, 1979.

Capute, A., Accardo, P., Vining, E., Rubeinstein, J., and Harryman, S. Primitive Reflex Profile. Monographs in Developmental Pediatrics, Vol. 1. Baltimore, University Park Press, 1978.

Casaer, P. Postural Behavior in Newborn Infants. Philadelphia, Lippincott, 1979.

Chandler, L. S., Andrews, M. S., and Swanson, M. W. Movement Assessment of Infants: A Manual. Rolling Bay, WA, 1980.

Erhardt, R. Erhardt Developmental Prehension Assessment. Ramsco Publ. Comp., Laurel, MD, 1982, rev. 1984.

Gesell, A., and Amatruda, C. S. Developmental Diagnosis. Normal and Abnormal Child Development. New York, Hoeber, 1947.

Haberfellner, H. Zur Frueherkennung Der Cerebralen Bewegungsstoerungen. *Oester Aerzt.* 32:1092-1095, 1977.

Hochleitner, M. Pathologische Motorische Entwicklung Bei Cerebralparese, Motoskopische Diagnostik. Goettingen, Institut fuer den Wissenschaftlichen Film, C 1107, 1973.

Illingworth, R. S. The Development of the Infant and Young Child, Normal and Abnormal, 3rd ed. London, Livingstone, 1967.

Ingram, T. T. S. The new approach to early diagnosis of handicaps in childhood. *Dev. Med. Child Neurol.* 11:279-290, 1969.

Koeng, E. Fruehdiagnose Cerebraler Laehmungen. *Paediatr. Fortbldg. Praxis* 1:37-44, 1962.

Koeng, E. Frueherfassung Cerebraler Bewegungsstoerungen. *Paediatr. Fortbldg. Praxs* 33:1-14, 1972.

Milani-Comparetti, A., and Gidoni, E. A. Pattern analysis of motor development and its disorders. *Dev. Med. Child Neurol.* 9:625-630, 1967.

Milani-Comparetti, A., and Gidoni, E. A. Routine development examination in normal and retarded children. *Dev. Med. Child Neurol.* 9:631-638, 1967.

Paine, R. S. Early recognition of neuromotor disabilities in infants with low birth weight. *Dev. Med. Child Neurol.* 11:455-459, 1969.

Peiper, A. Cerebral Function in Infancy and Childhood. New York, Consultants Bureau, 1963.

Prechtl, H., and Beintema, D. The Neurological Examination of the Full-Term Newborn Infant. Clinics in Developmental Medicine, No. 12. London, The Spastics Society Medical Education and Information Unit in association with Heinemann, 1964.

Rosenblith, J. F. Behavioral Examination of the Neonate. Proceedings from Comprehensive Management of Infants at Risk for CNS Deficit, May, 1974. Division of Physical Therapy, University of North Carolina, Chapel Hill, 1975.

Saint-Anne Dargassies, S. Neurodevelopmental symptoms during the first year of life. *Dev. Med. Child Neurol.* 14:235-246, 1972.

Saint-Anne Dargassies, S. Neurological Development in the Full-Term and Premature Neonate. Amsterdam, Elsevier, 1977.

Stern, F. The reflex development of the infant. *Am. J. Occup. Ther.* 25: 155-158, 1971.

Touwen B. Neurological Development in Infancy. Clinics in Developmental Medicine, No. 58. London, Heinemann, 1976.

Weisz, St. Studies in equilibrium reaction. *J. Nerv. Ment. Dis.* 88:150-162, 1938.

White, B. The First Three Years of Life. Englewood Cliffs, NJ, Prentice-Hall, 1975.

Wilson, J. Developmental reflex test. In Vulpe, S. (Ed.), The Vulpe Assessment Battery. National Institute on Mental Retardation, Toronto, 1977.

Wilson, J. Cerebral Palsy. In Campbell, S. (Ed.), Pediatric Neurologic Physical Therapy. Churchill Livingstone, New York, 1984.

6

Neurodevelopmental Assessment of Infants: Procedures

OVERVIEW

Examination and screening procedures preceding the therapy evaluation avail the therapist with some background information of the patient (see also Chaps. 2 and 3). When the diagnosis is not sufficiently clear, identification of suspect central nervous system (CNS) dysfunction and consequent referral for further assessment are based on some of the following symptoms.

1. Stereotyped behavior, paucity of movement, excessive and disorganized movement.
2. Poor control and alignment of head, face not in vertical plane, hyper-extension of head and neck
3. Consistent elevation of shoulder girdle, scapular protraction or retraction
4. Pronounced anterior or posterior pelvic tilt, incomplete hip extension
5. Hypotonicity with "frog posture" of limbs
6. Hypertonicity-inability to adapt to support surface or to active and passive movement
7. Low proximal tonus combined with high distal tonus, pronounced fisting of hands with pronation, and internal rotation of arms
8. Pronounced extensor patterns of legs with adduction of hips and clawing of toes
9. Feeding problems

The therapy assessment aims at analyzing in depth the quality of sensori-motor functions, adaptive and feeding behavior. A detailed analysis of normal and abnormal development is presented in Chapter 4. This chapter presents an interdisciplinary model for the therapy assessment; evaluates developmental skills and quality of underlying motor patterns; assesses adaptive behavior; describes a detailed feeding evaluation. Recommendations for an evaluation report and a motor evaluation form are also included.

For the assessment to be a meaningful tool for treatment and management, programming, it must go beyond a mere description of presented behavior. The therapist attempts to determine how different responses effect each other. It is important to find the primary component in a chain reaction of abnormal responses and to determine the most important postural mechanisms and motor components that would allow more appropriate function. The therapist should at all times be guided by the infant's behavior. Only then will the assessment be a truly investigative process and a helpful tool for designing a meaningful treatment program. Concepts and basic principles underlying this assessment approach are listed in Chapter 5.

INITIAL EVALUATION

Organization

Experts in different disciplines assess different sections of the infant's behavior. Better understanding of the total situation of patients and family mandates close communication between the different disciplines. Implementation of the team concept in the initial therapy assessment or screening seems preferable to separate evaluations by each specialist. Different models of the team approach are practiced and must be adjusted to the special circumstances. The therapy team includes physical, occupational, and speech therapists who collaborate closely with the physician, social worker, home service staff, psychologist, and teacher. At least one team member should evaluate the patient and family members in the home environment.

When the initial evaluation is carried out by a whole team, it will not be complete and detailed. The team aims to gather the most important information in each area of development: sensorimotor behavior, feeding, pre-speech, and language development, sensory functions, social, emotional, and cognitive development. The initial evaluation serves to determine major problems and areas requiring immediate intervention. Recommendations for further evaluation in specific areas will result from this.

The combined information of all team members outlines the infant's abilities and defines areas of concern, allowing the recommendations for intervention programs to be tailored to the individual needs of patient and family. This information must be presented to the family as soon as possible. The multidisciplinary team evaluation minimizes the time the family must wait for evaluation results.

Interviewing the Parent

At the start of the session, the team should obtain information from the accompanying parent about the infant's behavior at home, possible difficulties in care taking, the family's major concerns relative to the infant's deficits, and, finally, the family's expectations for their child's future.

Method of Assessment

The sensorimotor evaluation is carried out by observing spontaneous behavior, eliciting specific responses, and assessing the patient's potential for more mature postural reactions as facilitated through specific handling.

During the interview, the therapist establishes a rapport with both the parent and the infant. Interaction between the infant and the parent is observed as well as other adaptive behavior (see Chap. 5). Postural reactions to being carried and undressed are assessed. The parent is then asked to place the child on the mat for further observation of spontaneous behavior. Reactions to the separation from the parent, interest in and interaction with toys, as well as motor behavior are observed. Sensorimotor behavior is described as evidenced by motor functions and the quality of motor patterns as described in Chapter 5. Special emphasis is placed on righting reactions and equilibrium responses.

When placed on a mat, the infant is allowed to move without help and in this way to show whole movement repertoire without extensive prompting. Alternatively, the therapist sets up the environment by selectively placing toys around, thus challenging to the very limit, the child's available motor abilities and skills.

EVALUATION OF MOTOR DEVELOPMENT

Motor Behavior in Different Positions

Spontaneous motor functions and specific postural reactions are observed and elicited in a variety of positions. Special attention is focused on abnormal motor patterns which are repeated in various positions. Criteria for normal and abnormal sensorimotor behavior and some respective examples have been discussed in detail in Chapters 4 and 5. The limitations observed in spontaneous behavior are further investigated through selective handling following some of the procedures described below as applies to each case.

Supine

The extent and quality of spontaneous posture and movements are recorded before the therapist handles the infant.

Any predominant postural symmetry or asymmetry should be carefully evaluated. Asymmetrical posturing of the limbs is related to proximal patterns, namely, turning the head, posture of shoulder girdle, pelvis and trunk. Asymmetry of movements, such as reaching, grasping, kicking, and so on, is easy to detect.

Predominant extensor tonus is expressed in hyperlordosis of the cervical and lumbar spine, but also in scapular adduction and retraction of the arms. Elevation of the shoulders often accompanies poor head control. It should be noted if the head position determines body posture and oral posture or if the infant is able to differentiate movements of head, shoulder girdle, and trunk. Primitive or abnormal posture of the limbs, such as "frog position," is recorded.

Prevalence of static postures or the presence of movements such as hand-play, hands to feet, and their respective quality are described. Ability or disability to move out of the supine position is reported and the patterns used are noted (i.e., segmental rolling, primitive, total, or abnormal patterns). Some infants may use "bridging" and abnormal extension for progression while supine.

The therapist then handles the infant for a more precise assessment of postural tonus. The head position and its influence on the distribution of tonus are closely observed. Restrictions of mobility and contractures can be investigated at the same time. The infant's reactions to handling by the therapist are also interpreted as to tactile sensitivity.

Full overhead extension of the arms may be difficult to achieve and may cause excessive winging of the scapula and compensatory hyperlordosis of the lumbar spine. Mobility of the hips is tested. A symmetrical position of the pelvis must be ensured during these tests to determine accurately the range of mobility. Repetitive and brisk abduction of the hips may reveal underlying hypertonicity even when the basic tonus is low. Dorsiflexion of the ankle may be reduced due to abnormal extensor tonus. The degree of elongation of the neck can be evaluated by elevating pelvis and legs while elongating the spine. Head righting and active flexion against gravity are evaluated by pulling the infant by his or her hands to a sitting position except when head control is obviously poor.

An infant who does not spontaneously bring the hands together or to his or her mouth, feet, etc., is encouraged to reach with both hands for a toy held in midline. Assistance is given as required. Hearing and auditory attention are tested using a noise-making toy or by crumpling a piece of paper. A toy is also used to determine focusing and visual tracking ability. Toys of different textures are used to investigate tactile sensitivity.

Tracking may cause the infant to roll from supine to prone. Otherwise, the therapist facilitates rolling from the infant's pelvis while assessing whether proper head and trunk righting are applied.

Prone

The assessment in prone starts again with an observation of spontaneous posture and movements, such as reaching, rolling, and creeping. The degree and quality of extension against gravity is related to chronological age (see Chap. 4). If, during rolling toward prone, the infant's arms get stuck under his or her body, the therapist facilitates weight shifting from pelvis or trunk to allow the infant to free the arms. When the pull into flexion is strong, the therapist places the infant's arms forward for propping. This is a good opportunity to assess tonus and mobility of shoulder girdle and arms. Lateral righting, the ability to shift weight, and to reach for objects are evaluated in the puppy position and/or while propped on the hands. Assistance may be necessary to stabilize the pelvis in children lacking hip extension.

Using a toy, the therapist tries to elicit progression which can take the form of pivoting, while leaning on the hands, pushing backward (caudally) on extended arms, rolling, or creeping on the belly. Any distinct asymmetry (use of limbs, head position, torsion of trunk and pelvis) is recorded. The excessive use of arms, as in "commando crawling" (belly creeping) may result in tight extension and adduction of the legs. Where spontaneous belly crawling is not achievable, the therapist facilitates a shift of weight from trunk or pelvis to elicit the amphibian reaction. This function is preparatory for crawling; where abnormal tonus prevails, the infant will fail to achieve a sufficient degree of dissociation of movements.

Quadruped

When appropriate, chronologically and developmentally, the infant is encouraged to assume the quadruped position and to crawl on hands and knees. When balance and dissociation of movements are poor, both hips are kept in pronounced flexion during crawling, and more or less tight dorsiflexion of the ankle may be present. When the hypertonicity is strong, crawling takes the form of bunny hopping. Rotation and counterrotation between shoulder girdle and pelvis cannot occur as long as the spine is excessively flexed or extended and as long as the legs are in pronounced abduction. Upper extremity weight bearing is assessed for pronounced scapular protraction and elevation, internal rotation of shoulders, insufficient or excessive extension of the arms, and fisting of the hands. Any postural asymmetry is recorded.

Progression

Other forms of progression, such as rolling, belly crawling, etc., are evaluated for movement flow, postural alignment, and postural-functional symmetry.

Sitting

The sitting position and the ability to assume sitting are evaluated. Has the infant sufficient proximal stability to use the hands freely for manipulation? When necessary, minimal assistance is given by the examiner. The sitting posture is analyzed for postural alignment between pelvis, shoulder girdle, and head as viewed from the front (lateral flexion of the spine, lateral tilt of shoulder girdle and pelvis), from the side (flexion or extension of upper and/or lower trunk and hips, anterior or posterior pelvic tilt), and in the transverse plane (torsion of pelvis, shoulder girdle, and trunk, and turning of head). Does the infant sit on the ischial tuberosities or the sacrum? The posture of the lower extremities is evaluated for predominantly primitive (flexion, abduction, external rotation of hips, flexion of knees) abnormal (flexion, adduction, internal rotation of hips), or mature and differentiated patterns.

Are the feet used for patterns of fixation? Are the arms held in high guard posture? It should be recorded whether the arms are used for propping or whether they are free for manipulation; there may also be abnormal posturing of the upper extremities such as scapular protraction and elevation, internal rotation of the shoulders, and so on.

Symmetry of weight bearing on the hips is best evaluated by placing both hands under the patient's pelvis. Righting and equilibrium reactions as well as protective extension of the arms can be elicited while the therapist shifts the center of gravity to either side and backward or forward, either from the pelvis or from the trunk. Sitting balance and rotation within the body axis can also be elicited when the therapist encourages the infant to reach for toys in all directions, including backward. This may lead to a change of position from sitting to quadruped, side sitting, or prone. Degree of control and quality of movements are noted.

The infant who lacks trunk control and dissociation of movements often learns to sit unsupported by sitting between the heels and thus achieves a broad and stable base (W sitting). In these infants, sitting balance and posture are to be evaluated in longleg sitting as outlined above.

Upper Extremity Function

Activities of reaching, grasping, and releasing are evaluated as to accuracy, voluntary control, and refinement. Is tonus in the hands adaptable enough to properly contour hands to objects held? Is reaching accompanied by weight shifts through trunk and pelvis? Some children may achieve stability for release and manipulation of objects by leaning on the hand. Weight bearing and weight shifting are assessed in prone, quadruped, and sitting. In all positions, the therapist may manipulate the infant from pelvis and trunk to achieve the desired weight distribution. Protective extension can be tested in sitting and standing.

Standing and Walking

Abnormal patterns observed in lower positions may become even more pronounced when the child stands or walks. The emphasis of evaluation is on postural alignment, base of support, postural control, and the patterns of weight bearing and weight shifting. Some typical patterns of standing and walking have been described in Chapter 4.

Supported standing is assessed in the nonambulatory infant following the same criteria.

Elicited Primitive and Postural Reflexes

A test for positive and negative supporting as well as the parachute reaction of the legs can be combined with the test for lateral righting of head and trunk in vertical suspension. The Landau reaction is tested in ventral suspension.

The influence of the Moro reflex, where present, is usually noticeable during the evaluation and may, therefore, not require a specific test. Similarly, tonic reflex posturing and its interference with appropriate postural reactions is expressed in spontaneous behavior. A specific test for these reflexes may therefore be superfluous.

MOTOR EVALUATION REPORT

The therapist should record motor patterns in as much detail as possible to identify consistent and dominant abnormal reactions. For a clear and meaningful report, however, this information must be condensed, categorized, and interpreted. Chapter 5 contains suggestions on how to categorize behavior. The therapist's interpretation of major and primary deficiencies determines emphasis of treatment and management plan. Recommendations for intended programming should also be included.

When the report is kept in a descriptive format, a consistent outline should be followed at each subsequent reevaluation to allow a comparison. A checklist evaluation form may narrow the observation to the items listed while overlooking some of the infant's most important behaviors. Checklists also make it difficult to investigate how different behaviors correlate with each other on an individual basis. The Motor Evaluation Form presented here (see Appendix) is intended as a guide, leaving room for adaptations to the individual needs of each patient.

EVALUATION OF ORAL DEVELOPMENT AND FEEDING SKILLS

This part of the evaluation consists of: a brief postural assessment as it relates to oral function, an analysis of feeding patterns, and an oral examination.

Postural Assessment

Postural reactions which influence feeding skills include the degree and quality of head control, trunk control, and shoulder girdle posture; the quality, adaptibility, and distribution of postural tonus; and posturing in tonic reflex patterns.

These postural reactions can be, to a great extent, assessed while the infant is still on the parent's lap. The alignment between head, shoulders, and pelvis should be described and related to oral and facial posture. Retraction of head and shoulders, or abnormal and dominating extension throughout the body, or lack of stability through the spine, are often accompanied by open mouth posture, abnormal tongue posture, drooling, and, possibly, retraction of the lips. Abnormal flexor tonus may underlie lip pursing and tightly closed jaws. Consistent postural and oral asymmetry should be noted. The therapist observes whether the infant puts hands or objects into the mouth.

This postural assessment can be combined with an interview of the parent about feeding procedures and difficulties. The parent is asked about the usual feeding position, types and approximate amount of food consumed, types of utensils used, and the length of the feeding procedure.

To allow a more detailed and qualitative assessment of feeding behavior, the parent is asked to feed the infant.

Observation of Feeding Patterns

Position

While the parent feeds the infant, the therapist notes the infant's position and possible impact on the oral function. Is the infant reclined, and how far? Or is the baby seated upright? Alignment of head, trunk, and pelvis, and obvious tightness in the shoulder girdle and neck area are documented. Are patterns of abnormal extension or asymmetry reinforced by the infant's position or by the parent's approach? How much support is given to the spine, to the head, and is it sufficient?

Sucking

Sucking is analyzed for efficiency, loss of liquid, and coordination between sucking, swallowing, and breathing. The movement patterns of jaw, tongue, and lips are also observed.

Normally developing infants progress through three different stages of sucking behavior. The neonate approximates the lips tightly around the nipple. Due to this seal, the rhythmical raising and lowering of tongue and jaw create negative pressure in the oral cavity which assists in emptying the nipple. A decrease of flexor tonus and a relative increase of extensor tonus reduce this tight approximation around the nipple soon thereafter. The baby then relies mostly on the suckling pattern where the nipple is stroked with tongue movements of protraction and retraction. With increased postural stability and better coordination between patterns of flexion and extension, the baby is again able to create good lip sealing and a negative pressure to suck on the nipple with controlled upward and downward movements of the tongue.

Abnormally developing infants seem to maintain a suckling pattern for a prolonged time. This is combined with an abnormal swallowing pattern in which the tongue protrudes between the lips and pushes the liquid out.

For infants who are bottle fed, the type of nipple, ease of liquid flow, and consistency of liquid are described.

Cup Drinking

The pattern of cup drinking changes during normal development. While initial attempts at about five months of age still reflect a sucking pattern, increased lip action gradually transforms the sucking action into a sipping motion. Traces of sucking behavior are seen in children up to two years of age and are expressed in a pattern of "chewing on the cup." This is overcome when the child achieves a high degree of dissociation of jaw, tongue, and lip movements, allowing good jaw stabilization.

Abnormally developing children often apply primitive or abnormal sucking patterns to cup drinking. Frequently, the cup is placed too far into the mouth, aggravating lip retraction and/or biting on the cup.

As well as evaluating the drinking pattern, the therapist should note the size of the cup and the liquid used.

Spoon Feeding

As with cup drinking, the young infant uses sucking patterns when starting to take food from the spoon, making initial attempts at spoon feeding messy. In the latter months of the first year, the infant gradually develops the ability to remove the food from the spoon with the lips. With intrinsic movements, the tongue gathers the food into a bolus, transfers it back to be swallowed, and leans against the alveolar ridge during swallowing to seal off the oral cavity preventing food from escaping.

A primitive or abnormal suck interferes with successful spoon feeding. Instead of taking the food off the spoon with the lips, the tongue thrusts forward and the lips retract. Scraping the food along the teeth or gums further reinforces retraction of the lips. During swallowing, the tongue may protrude and push food out. The hypersensitive infant may bite down on the spoon in an uncontrolled tonic motion. Hyperextension of the jaw may occur in response to the approaching spoon. When dealing with severe feeding and swallowing problems, some parents may resort to "bird feeding," that is, the infant's head is tilted far back and the food is dropped into the throat, thus the infant gets no sensory input for actively removing the food from the spoon, nor for transferring the food back with the tongue to be swallowed (Fig. 1).

The therapist should also note the type and shape of the spoon as well as which food is presented to the infant.

Biting and Chewing

The development of biting and chewing begins before the infant has acquired molars. By about 6 to 7 months of age, when the infant has gained good

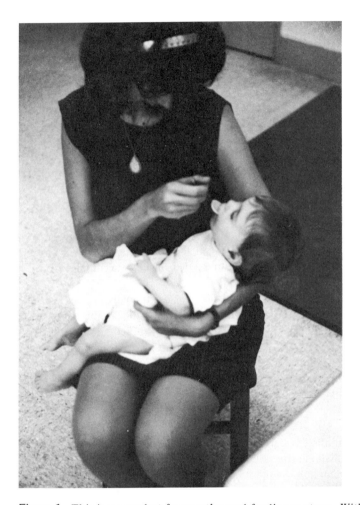

Figure 1 This is a poor but frequently used feeding posture. With the head tilted so far back into extension, it is very difficult to achieve mouth closure and proper swallowing patterns. Instead of the tongue transferring the food back, the food glides back by gravity ("bird feeding"). This feeding position does not allow the infant to develop mature and controlled feeding patterns. (From *The Infant with Cerebral Palsy: An Approach to Identification, Management, and Treatment.* A. L. Scherzer. Private printing, New York, 1973.)

head control and some trunk stability is attained, the infant starts to take
solid food for chewing. At that time, the primitive up and down movement
of the bite reflex is modified. For biting, the mandible moves forward while
the jaw opens, and slides backward along and behind the upper gums or teeth
to tear off a piece of food. With the emergence of tongue lateralization, the
food is then transported to the chewing surface and is fenced there between
tongue and cheek during the chewing action. Gradually, the chewing motion
incorporates a rotary component. After the food has been sufficiently
ground and moistened with saliva, the tongue moves it posteriorly to be swallowed. Primitive sucking and biting reflexes are suppressed and the gag reflex
decreases and is no longer elicited from the frontal third of the oral cavity.
Persistence of infantile feeding reflexes inhibits lateralization of the tongue
and the development of rotary movements of the jaw. As a consequence, the
food cannot be brought to and held on the biting surface. Instead, it is
maintained in the mouth until it is softened and can be sucked down. Frequently, much of the food is pushed out by the tongue or accumulates on the
palate.

During the assessment of biting and chewing, the therapist focuses on the
presence of mature, dissociated oral movements or on the dominance of reflex behavior and abnormal swallowing patterns. Disturbed oral function
may also lead to frequent choking on food. Vomiting during or soon after
feeding is another problem which requires attention because it interferes
with the infant's nourishment and may present a real danger because of possible aspiration of vomitus.

Self-Feeding

When solid food intake is started, the infant also begins to fingerfeed. The
lack of refined manipulative skills at this stage causes babies to push the
food from the palm into the mouth rather than using a controlled placement
with their fingers. By 15 to 18 months, the baby is able to handle a cup and
a spoon with some help and supervision, and by 2 years of age, the child can
handle food with moderate spilling.

Infants with CNS impairment may show a significant developmental delay in this area. Lack of sufficient head control and poor trunk and shoulder
girdle stability require that the arms be used for support. The child who
can free his or her arms but is restricted to total patterns fails to achieve
graded supination of the forearm while approaching the mouth. In the last
phase, the spoon or cup must be held stable while the head moves forward
and the lips grab utensil and food. The handicapped child may not reach
this level of motor control. In fingerfeeding, the infant may not be able to

hold the food between the fingers; release may only be possible when leaning the hand against the face, thus pushing the food into the mouth in a primitive or abnormal fashion. When evaluating self-feeding, it is important to note whether the effort involved results in abnormal facial and oral tonus.

Observation of a feeding session also gives a general impression of the interaction between parent and infant, their degree of tension, and their way of coping with any difficulties.

Oral Examination

This aspect of the evalution permits a selective and systematic investigation of those oral functions which seem to underlie the disturbed feeding behavior as displayed during the feeding session. The information obtained through the oral examination should give the therapist a more complete understanding of the patient's oral development.

A relaxed, comfortable, and symmetrical position must be chosen. Examining the infant in different positions may reveal different aspects of the abnormality of oral responses, and may help to determine the optimal function.

The oral examination includes:

Description of oral posture, tonus, and structure
Description of oral sensitivity to selective sensory stimuli
Test for oral reflexes
An assessment of vegetative breathing as it relates to swallowing and
   feeding

Posture, Tonus, and Structure

As in the postural evaluation, the oral examination starts with an observation of spontaneous posture and movement. Some of this information was already gathered while the infant was still on the parent's lap. However, a different picture may be presented when the baby is well positioned and optimally supported.

Posture and tonus of cheeks, lips, and tongue should be evaluated at rest, during different stages of excitement, and during function, for example, during vocalization. The examiner should record manidibular posture and movements for protraction, retraction, depression, and lateral deviation. In addition to a possible asymmetry of the jaw, there may also be asymmetrical posturing of the tongue. It is noted whether spontaneous jaw and lip closure is present, or whether the mouth is kept open and the infant is drooling. The degree of grading of oral movements is described.

Abnormal tonus is expressed in facial and oral motions. Hypertonicity is reflected in a lack of facial and oral movements. The lips are tense and often retracted, the tongue may be retracted or elevated. The hypertonic tongue may also be elongated and thrust forward with a pointed tip. The hypotonic infant is characterized by a paucity of facial expressions, but the posture differs. Cheeks and lips are floppy, the tongue is flat and broad, and rests either on the floor of the mouth or interdentally. Fluctuations of tonus and involuntary movements create exaggerated grimacing which is typical of the athetoid patient.

For a more accurate evaluation of oral tonus, the examiner places one finger between cheeks and gums, as well as between lips and gums and touches the tongue to feel the degree of tension. It must be considered that touching the perioral and oral area provides a strong stimulus, possibly leading to a substantial increase of tonus. Also, it may not be acceptable to all patients and a resistance towards the intrusive touch by a stranger must be respected.

For the intraoral examination, a facial grasp for adequate control of the infant's mandibular movements is recommended. A detailed description of the different facial grasps can be found in Chapter 7 (Jaw Control).

The condition of the gums should be observed initially. Hyperplasia and swollen gums are often present in infants taking anticonvulsive medication. A description of the occlusion and condition of the teeth follows. Tongue thrusting and abnormal sucking patterns contribute to malocclusions, such as open bite, overbite, and cross bite. These, in turn, may aggravate abnormal biting and chewing patterns. The condition and shape of teeth are frequently impaired in combination with severe tongue thrusting and abnormal sucking patterns.

Hard and soft palates are examined for gross deviations which may influence food intake. An extremely narrow, high arched palate does not provide sufficient room to house the tongue which consequently rests interdentally. The abnormal tongue position interferes with normal patterns of swallowing, where the tongue leans against the alveolar ridge. The normal position of the tongue against the alveolar ridge seems to form a stimulating force for the maintenance of the proper arch width in the maxilla. Structure and tonus of the soft palate affect swallowing. Abnormal tonus or congenital malformations, such as cleft palate, may affect sucking and swallowing. When, during swallowing, the soft palate is not moved into apposition with the posterior wall of the pharynx to seal off the nasal cavity, food or liquid may escape to the nasal passages and aspiration may occur.

Sensitivity

Sensory stimuli within and around the mouth elicit a chain reaction of feeding reflexes in the normal infant. Efficient feeding behavior depends on and is regulated by accurate oral sensory feedback. The hypersensitive child reacts to stimuli of touch, taste, smell, and temperature with abnormal tension of lips, cheeks, and tongue. Retraction of the head and abnormal extension throughout the body may follow.

Deficiency of sensory feedback impairs oral function and needs close investigation. Observation of the feeding process reveals how the infant reacts to different stimuli. To appreciate more subtle tonal changes, the therapist selectively touches the oral and perioral area.

Reflexes

Perioral and oral touch also represent the stimulus for different oral reflexes. The reflexes to be tested are the rooting, suck-swallowing, bite, and gag reflexes.

The rooting reflex is present at birth and allows the infant to move the head in search of food long before head control is established. As a stimulus, the infant is stroked on the cheeks and above and below the lips. The reflex is positive when the infant pouts lips, protrudes tongue, and turns the head in the direction of the stimulus. In the infant with CNS impairment, the rooting reflex may be particularly pronounced, inhibiting more selective lip action and contributing to asymmetries of lips, jaw, and tongue.

Associated with the rooting reflex is the suck-swallowing reflex which is elicited when a finger or nipple is brought into the mouth. A description of this reflex is discussed in the section "Observation of Feeding Patterns." At this point the therapist determines whether sucking is a voluntary response or a reflexive behavior.

The bite reflex is also present during the early months of life and is elicited by touching the gums to the side or on the biting surface. The infant reacts with a straight upward-downward movement of the mandible. In normal development, this reflex behavior is altered by the emergence of mature biting and chewing. In abnormal development, the bite reflex is easily elicited and may persist, interfering with the development of mature biting and chewing. Instead of eliciting a phasic and continuous biting motion, touch of the gums may elicit a tonic and uncontrolled bite in infants with CNS dysfunction; release of the bite is often difficult.

The gag reflex is elicited by touching the posterior part of the tongue or palate. This protective reflex is present at birth. When the infant starts to chew on solids, the area sensitive to the gag reflex is gradually reduced and restricted to the posterior part of the oral cavity. In the neurologically impaired infant, the gag reflex is often hyperactive, especially in combination with swallowing problems. Absence of this protective reaction, also connected with CNS dysfunction, poses a hazard and needs to be considered when feeding the infant.

Breathing Patterns

Successful manipulation of food requires coordination between feeding and breathing, since the pharynx forms the passage for both food intake and respiration. Swallowing is alternative and dominant over respiration (Doty and Bosma). In the suckling infant, the rhythm of both breathing and swallowing is influenced and directed by the sucking center (Peiper). In the neurologically impaired infant, the interaction between sucking, breathing, and swallowing may be disorganized, which can lead to choking and aspiration.

The infant should be described as either a nose breather or mouth breather. In normal development, the infant must breathe through the nose until 3 months of age. The infant with CNS deficit often relies on mouth breathing, which increases the danger of swallowing air and of aspiration. Since nasal respiration requires approximation between tongue and soft palate, a motor disturbance in these areas may contribute to patterns of abnormal breathing.

After reviewing and correlating the information gathered during the postural assessment, feeding, and oral examination, the therapist concludes the report with recommendations for appropriate intervention.

APPENDIX MOTOR EVALUATION

Name: Chart no.:   Birth date: Date: Therapist:

I. General impressions (alertness, interaction with parent/environment, communication, reaction to stimuli):

II. Sensory deficits and other pertinent medical information:

III. The motor functions listed below are assessed as to their postural adaptations (normal or abnormal) in the positions that are appropriate for the patient.

Motor functions	Motor patterns: Normal postural adaptations	Abnormal postural responses

1. Observation of spontaneous behavior: positional control, UE skills, transitions, progression, ADL, oromotor function, communication	1. Righting against gravity
	    extension
	    flexion
	    lateral flexion
	    axial rotation
		1. Sinks into gravity
		2. Pushes into support
		3. Obligatory asymmetry
		4. Hyperextension of head and neck

2. Elicit specific reactions if not displayed spontaneously:
    righting
    rolling
    transitions
    Landau reaction
    equilibrium
    protective extension
	2. Head control
	    face vertical
	    mouth horizontal
	    neck elongated
	    (after 4 mos)
		5. Persistent shoulder girdle protraction/retraction
		6. Pronounced anterior/posterior pelvic tilt
		7. Stereotyped patterns (frog position)

3. Test for mobility and postural tonus	3. Symmetry, midline control (after 4 mos) 4. Shoulder girdle aligned on stable trunk (after 4 mos in well-supported positions)	8. Paucity/excess of movement 9. Lack of mobility

APPENDIX (Continued)

    5. Differentiation and variation of movements
    6. Postural stability and mobility
       equilibrium reactions
       protective extension of
         arms (starting at 6 mo)

IV. Overall quality of motor behavior (variability, grading, sequencing)
V. Predominant motor patterns
VI. Restricted mobility, (risk for) contractures, deformities
VII. Reaction to sensory stimulation (kinesthetic, tactile, proprioceptive, auditory, visual)
VIII. Additional comments
IX. Summary
    Displayed behaviors seem to be typical—if not give apparent reason
X. Program goals
IX. Recommended procedures

7

Home Management

The immediate environment of an infant is controlled and represented by the family who determines to a great extent whether the infant will reach full physical, intellectual, and emotional potentialities. The quality of stimuli provided by the family shapes early learning. Initially, babies depend mostly on their mother to provide these early learning situations through her attention while feeding and caring for them, playing and communicating with them. The success of the infant in achieving continued independence and control over actions and the environment depends on how the parents relate and interact with the child.

While the infant's behavior is affected by the family, the family's behavior toward the infant is shaped by the infant's responses. Disturbed behavior resulting from central nervous system (CNS) dysfunction can inhibit interaction between infant and family. A lack of responsiveness or irritable behavior in an infant is likely to decrease the family's desire to play and interact with him or her. When abnormal postural reactions make handling difficult, the infant may be held and cuddled infrequently. When such tasks as feeding or bathing the infant represent a struggle on the mother's part, social interaction is likely to be omitted during these activities and feedback to the baby is scarce and negative. The baby with poor control of posture and movement is furthermore seldom encouraged to assist and participate to full capability, however limited, in activities of dressing and feeding. As a consequence, the child may become more and more passive and dependent, and lack of interaction deprives the handicapped infant of experiences normal babies are exposed to, which may further retard and disturb development.

In addition to the reduced frequency of handling and interaction, the infant with motor disturbances is often carried, dressed, fed, etc. in an abnormal fashion because the parent adapts to the baby's aberrant reactions. Constant repetition reinforces these abnormal reactions and in time they become firmly established, posing a severe obstacle to the learning of new and more complex skills.

The emotional impact on the family caused by severe delay and disturbance of development can be detrimental to both the infant and the family. Difficulties in meeting the most vital needs of a baby often cause severe frustration and anxiety in a parent; a feeling of inadequacy and even resentment may emerge. Appropriate counseling must aim at alleviating such destructive reactions. Early intervention for home management should be a high priority in every infant program. The therapist must help parents to find the most efficient way of handling and caring for their infant. Parents must be educated and trained in how to behave appropriately to help reinforce and maximize the infant's skills while continuing to feel adequate in their own role as parents.

Advice in home management is tailored to the individual needs of each patient as well as his or her family. Instructions in specific handling techniques are most effective when they can be carried out in the patient's home. The parent who is taught basic concepts of normal and abnormal development and who understands general principles of intervention is better equipped to generalize handling techniques to accommodate a variety of situations. Parents should be taught which postures are conducive to different movements and which severely limit or inhibit motor activities. One way in which parents may learn about limitations of movements is to experience the effects of these limitations on themselves during training sessions.

Group sessions for parents are another way to present this information. The social aspect of parent groups is a further bonus of this type of parent training: the opportunity for sharing experiences and feelings with parents of other handicapped infants can be extremely valuable and supportive. Parent-infant sessions, on the other hand, are best carried out on an individual basis.

This chapter addresses home management on a general, conceptual basis, describes normal and abnormal postures which accompany motor functions of home management, and gives some samples of specific handling techniques. It does not include recommendations for fostering language, perceptual, and cognitive skills.

POSITIONING AND SEATING

A major concern of the management program is proper positioning and seating to allow the infant to function to optimal potential during play activities and feeding.

The family is faced with considerable problems in seating the severely impaired infant who lacks head and trunk control. The baby who lacks sufficient extension against gravity is not able to raise the head when prone and prop on elbows or hands. These infants, then, usually spend the day lying supine. Without sufficient flexion against gravity this position is very restrictive and hypotonic as well as hypertonic infants are quite inactive when they lie straight on their back. The abnormal postural tonus makes it difficult or impossible to raise the head and/or the legs for any active body exploration and for investigation of the surroundings. Without control against gravity the infant cannot roll toward the side or toward prone but is locked into the supine position. If the shoulders are retracted, the child cannot bring the hands together, preventing them or objects from reaching the mouth for stimulation and investigation. Resulting limitations of sensorimotor experiences and reduced interaction with the environment contribute to perceptual impairment, delay of body awareness, disturbance of body image, and the problem of tactile hypersensitivity, especially in the oral area.

Better positioning becomes a high priority. However, it must be stressed that there is no one optimal or ideal position for the developmentally delayed infant. It is important to foster postural control in a *variety of positions*. The infant who cannot change positions without assistance, should be repositioned frequently and must be provided with optimal (not maximal) support in each position.

When adaptive equipment is used, it must be observed that its purpose is to help patients *function at their best* rather than pursuing perfect alignment while immobilizing the patient with straps and adaptations. Function does not require perfect alignment. Setting realistic goals and expectations is as important for selecting adaptive equipment as it is for treatment.

Supine Position

NORMAL DEVELOPMENT

Early play activities and initial manual and oral investigations take place in supine. Relatively high flexor tonus already affords the newborn some antigravity postures and movements in supine. More controlled and deliberate patterns of flexion, however, start to evolve at about 3 months of age when the baby assumes a more symmetrical posture with the head predominantly in midline position. This is a prerequisite for bringing hands together and for engaging in hand to feet, feet to mouth, and other exploratory activities. By 5 and 6 months, control against gravity in supine has progressed so that the baby is able to lift head unassisted. The primitive total patterns of flexion are gradually differentiated and are combined with components of extension and rotation providing the infant, finally, with the ability to move out of the supine position unassisted into sidelying, prone, or sitting.

ABNORMAL DEVELOPMENT

Abnormal postural tonus interferes with control against gravity and causes the infant to sink or to push into the support. Optimal positioning and support are required to foster proper control against gravity.

Normal and abnormal motor patterns occurring in supine are described in detail in the section on "Postural Control in Supine," Chapter 4.

Positioning. Since turning the head to one side encourages extension, orientation of toys and other stimuli should stress midline position of the head when patterns of extension and asymmetry are predominant. Support of the head, shoulders, and upper trunk in a slightly flexed position allows the infant to bring arms forward and to keep the head in midline. For play activities the parent is shown how to help the baby lift the legs in an early pattern of flexion, abduction, or external rotation. Pelvis and trunk may have to be stabilized at the same time. A ribbon or a bell fastened around the ankle draws attention to the legs and feet and stimulates flexion and midline orientation.

Equipment. A slightly flexed supine position can be achieved when wedges or pillows are placed under the head and/or legs. Flexion of hips is also encouraged by propping the baby over an inflated tube, or by being placed in a hammock. Depending on the size of the netting, a lining may be required to prevent fingers or limbs from becoming entangled. Elevation of either end modifies the pattern and degree of flexion. Toys can be strung on stands or above the crib. Correct placement of the toys is essential for proper neck elongation and to enable the infant to reach them with the hands or to kick them with the feet. Frequently, toys are positioned directly above the head instead of further caudal as they should be to encourage neck elongation and tucking of the chin.

Prone Position

Babies develop independent postural control first in prone. This process is inititated with the development of head control, which in prone is achieved by four months of age. By five months, the infant can push up on both hands while prone. By six months, the infant has developed equilibrium reactions and between six to eight months, full extensor control is demonstrated in the Landau reaction.

The infant who demonstrates abnormal progravity extension in supine should be frequently positioned in prone in order to develop greater normal antigravity extension. The parent must be instructed in the correct postures which make lifting the head and propping on the arms possible. Normal and abnormal motor patterns occurring in prone are described in detail in Chapter 4, section on "Postural Control in Prone."

Positioning. With the pelvis off the supporting surface, much of the body weight rests on the upper trunk which limits the degree to which the infant can raise the head. Hip extension is necessary to stabilize the pelvis on the supporting surface. When the legs are widely abducted as in the typical "frog" position, hip extension cannot take place. The legs must, therefore, be placed in a pattern of extension and slight abduction of the hips. If necessary, sandbags or bolsters are placed alongside the legs to maintain proper positioning.

During upper extremity weight bearing, scapular protraction and internal rotation of the shoulder can be reduced when elbows are placed somewhat forward in relation to the shoulders. The parent is shown how to correct protraction and elevation of the scapula with one hand placed across clavicula, shoulder, and scapula while bringing the infant's arm forward with external rotation of the shoulder. Some support alongside the arms, for example, sandbags or bolsters, keeps the arms in proper position. Prone on elbows or hands is a very tiring position and is never maintained for long periods. The handicapped infant also should not be propped on elbows for an extended time. Instead, positioning in prone should make it possible for the infant to push up on hands or elbows when ready. Upper extremity weight bearing occurs also when the infant lies flat on the support with the shoulders fully flexed and the arms overhead. This position increases mobility between scapula and arm and is a good sensory preparation for upper extremity function.

Equipment. Placing the infant on an incline, such as provided by a foam wedge, may facilitate extension of the spine. For security and to facilitate hip extension, a restrainer can be used across the hips. The use of a roll or rolled towel to support and elevate the chest may cause the infant to pull the shoulders into extension and internal rotation against it which should be corrected.

Side-Lying Position

The side-lying position elicits lateral righting of head and trunk, and dissocia-
tin of motor patterns which leads to a pattern of overall extension on the
weight-bearing side and a pattern of overall flexion on the non-weight-bearing side (amphibian reaction). This degree of postural control is achieved normally by 5 to 6 months. The infant with problems of postural control rarely
assumes side lying. Nevertheless, the infant with dominant progravity flexion
and/or extension probably has a better chance to posturally organize when
lying on side.

Positioning. Proper postural alignment must be ensured. Undue extension
must be corrected, the trunk should be straight or slightly flexed and not
arched into extension, the head must be well-aligned with the trunk. Proper
placement of toys encourages flexion of neck and head. A pillow under the
head is used to properly align head and trunk. Both legs are flexed to provide
a broad base of support. When necessary, a pillow maintains the flexed position. Both arms are brought forward. The infant should, of course, be positioned on each side alternately.

Equipment. The infant who cannot remain in a side-lying position, and rolls
unintentionally and uncontrolledly toward supine or prone is supported by a
bolster in the back. When more support is needed, a stuffed animal or a sand-
bag can be placed in front of the chest. For classroom use it is convenient to
build a side-lying board that can be tilted into different angles from the horizontal.

Sitting Position

NORMAL DEVELOPMENT
The newborn attempts to align the head vertically in sitting, but, due to biomechanical and tonal conditions, the spine is flexed, so that the back is
slightly and evenly rounded. A 4-month-old infant can sit supported with
fairly good head control. Although a 6-month-old infant sits unsupported
for brief moments, the sitting posture indicates that trunk control is not yet
fully developed, increased adduction of the scapulae and "high guard" position of the arms compensate for the flexion of the lower part of the spine.
By 9 to 10 months the trunk is stable during unsupported sitting, the back
is straight, and the arms come down. Now, sitting balance is completed and
the baby is able to pivot and to reach in all directions, although these activities may still produce traces of unilateral "high guard" posturing.

ABNORMAL DEVELOPMENT

The infant with developmental delay requires support for a considerably longer time and to a much greater degree. Nevertheless, the infant should not be deprived of the opportunity to view the environment from a sitting position. However, even when well-supported, the infant with poor head and/or trunk control who has not yet developed extension of the lumbar spine should only sit for short periods at a time. Normal and abnormal development are further described in detail in the section on "Postural Control in Sitting," Chapter 4.

Positioning. The following postural components should be applied regardless of which and how much support is given. The hips must be flexed sufficiently to have the infant sit square on the buttocks, which allows the pelvis to be upright and the lumbar spine to be extended. Weight bearing must be symmetrical on both hips and thighs. The alignment between shoulders and the hips determines head and trunk posture, perpendicular alignment in the sagittal plane requires good integration between flexion and extension. When the shoulders are forward of the hips, the infant has to use extension to counteract gravity; when the shoulders are behind the hips, flexion is encouraged to overcome gravity. A slight degree of flexion, especially of the head, is desirable.

Equipment. A slightly reclined seat encourages the infant to lean against the back of the chair and tilt the head slightly forward. The angle between seat and back support is kept at 90 degrees. In order to achieve a straight back, the lumbar spine may require additional support.

The infant who shows a tendency to push into extension and to slide forward in the chair is ideally seated with flexed knees. In this case, the depth of the seat must be adjusted so that the knees can be comfortably bent while the infant sits all the way back in the seat; when the seat is too deep, the hips can be pushed easily into extension. A padded back panel can be inserted to adjust the depth of a highchair. Elevation of the seat in the front encourages the infant to slide all the way back. A nonslippery surface also reduces the danger of sliding forward. A belt across the thighs helps to stabilize the legs as a base of support while pelvis, trunk, and arms move.

A laptray or table gives security and provides a base for toys. A lip around the tray prevents objects from sliding off. When the chair is reclined, the angle of the tray may have to be tilted too.

When head and trunk control are very poor, lateral support is attached to the back of the chair enveloping both shoulders and preventing retraction of the arms. Lateral support for hips and legs provides symmetry and prevents marked abduction of the hips. Triangle chairs are widely used when trunk control is poor, although they provide good lateral support, the support to the low back must be evaluated to ensure proper extension of the back.

The head position is extremely important and needs special consideration. Any tendency to hyperextend the neck should be discouraged. An upright pelvis and good contact between thighs and support surface are often sufficient for achieving a normal head posture. When additional head support is indicated, it should be shaped according to the form of the head; a straight extension of the back panel pushes the head too much into flexion in an upright chair and can be very uncomfortable. Footrests must be reached comfortably. The footrest for a reclined seat should be appropriately tilted to discourage pronounced plantar-flexion.

For the infant with poor sitting balance it is often advisable to build a supportive seat insert which can be used in a highchair, chair, and carseat. When such a seat insert is used exclusively, it should be made adjustable to provide a variety of sitting postures. Infant seats with adjustable seat depth and angle of recline and with lateral support to trunk and hips are available commercially.

Equipment such as baby swings and highchairs usually fail to provide postural stability: they often require specially designed attachments or inserts following the concepts described above. Poor posture is also displayed in baby jumpers and baby walkers, which are favorites for infants and parents because they provide the baby with some mobility. Parents must be made aware that "standing" and "walking" without proper support and consequently with poor postural alignment do not teach the baby how to balance. On the contrary, they aggravate abnormal tonus and postures throughout the body and may reinforce structural deformities of feet and hips. This equipment is widely advertised to be used at a very early age (four months), which is earlier than an infant's motor and structure ability will allow the child to stand for long periods of time.

Independent Sitting

The infant who sits independently may also need some monitoring of sitting posture. When sitting on the floor, the hypotonic infant often spreads the legs in wide abduction. This wide base poses little challenge for balancing and does not encourage movement and postural changes. Parents are advised to reposition the baby's legs and gradually decrease the degree of abduction. Placement of toys all around the baby elicits balance and protective reactions.

Sitting on the floor in "W" position (sitting between the heels) is frequently seen in handicapped children; it may be functional for a short time
but it restricts the development of balance reactions and may lead to contractures when used excessively. Therefore, other positions should be encouraged
as often as feasable.

Car Safety Seats and Strollers

Principles described above also apply to the selection of car safety seats and
strollers. Contoured seats with snuggly fitting lateral trunk supports work
best when head and trunk control is a problem. Some carriages may only
work after a supportive seat insert is attached. The umbrella stroller has
found wide use for infants with a tendency to push into extension; however,
the lack of a firm back support reinforces pronounced flexion of the lumbar
spine and interferes with good trunk and head position. Strollers which are
adapted specifically for the handicapped infant but can nevertheless be folded
easily are commercially available; adaptations include trunk support, head
support, and thigh separator.

With any model of car safety seat or stroller, a seat belt across the hips se-
cures the infant in the seat; for this purpose the seat belt must cross the hips
diagonally. Too often it is attached to the back panel instead of the seat and
thus holds the infant across the abdomen which does not prevent him or her
from sliding forward underneath it. If additional support around the trunk is
needed, a second belt can be added.

Standing with Support

NORMAL DEVELOPMENT
Supported standing seems to please babies at a very early age. The 4-month-
old may try to stand on feet when helped to a sitting position. The ability to
pull to standing unassisted emerges during the last months of the first year
when the baby begins to acquire balance in the upright position.

ABNORMAL DEVELOPMENT
The handicapped infant also enjoys the upright position but needs substantially more support and guidance to achieve correct postural alignment so as
to develop a sense of balance.

Normal and abnormal patterns of standing are discussed in detail in the
section on "Patterns of Standing" in Chapter 4.

Positioning. Standing balance can be encouraged while the child leans
against a coffee table, sofa, or chair. It is important that the center of gravity

is well aligned over the base of support. Frequently, help is needed to bring pelvis and hips far enough forward. Hip extension and upright posture is facilitated when the feet are placed very close to the furniture which is used for support. External rotation of hips and eversion of feet broaden the base and may increase stability but interfere with weight shifting and balancing. The infant should therefore also be encouraged to stand with the feet straightforward.

Equipment. Prone boards, which are available commercially, and supine boards are helpful for the infant who still cannot pull to a standing position during the second or third year. Their support can be adjusted for a wide range of balancing skills: as freestanding units or to be placed against a table or kitchen counter.

Standing tables and infant walkers are only support mechanisms and offer little possibility for selective correction of posture. Without correct postural alignment, standing may be more detrimental rather than helpful; abnormal postures resulting from poor support during standing may range from poor head posture to distorted foot alignment. Poor foot alignment and abnormal patterns of weight bearing often result in pronounced adduction, flexion, and internal rotation of the hips, which severely interfere with the development of standing balance. The effects of these postural maladjustments may, in time, also be seen in other positions and may impair previously developed skills.

For proper alignment in standing, the hips must be brought into extension. On the prone board hip extension is ensured with a belt across the hip joints (Fig. 1a and b); when the hip belt is attached too high, the child sinks into flexion. On the supine board a belt across the thighs is often sufficient depending on the angle in which the board is reclined (see Fig. 2a and b). Otherwise, an additional belt is used across the lower rib cage. Foot placement determines the base of support; the hips should be slightly abducted and in slight external or neutral rotation. Pronounced external rotation or marked abduction result in weight bearing on the medial border of the foot.

Good weight distribution throughout the foot must be stressed and standing on the toes in plantar flexion is to be corrected. In case of structural foot deformities, the use of appropriate shoe inserts is indicated. If this option is not available, wedging of the footrest accomodates abnormal supination of the forefoot which can be a cause for excessive forefoot pronation in standing.

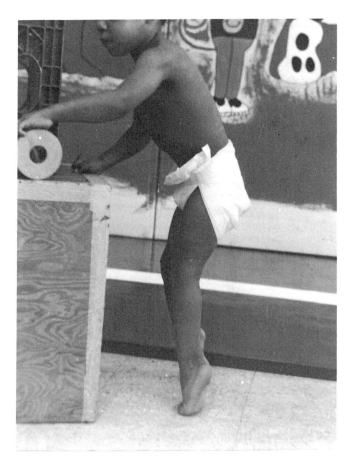

Figure 1a During the second year of life the handicapped child enjoys pulling to standing, although he or she may lack the appropriate motor control. As a result, posture and tonus become increasingly abnormal.

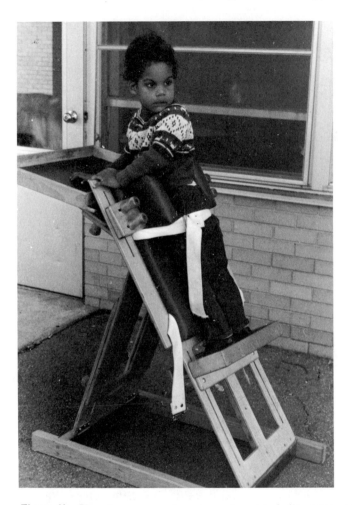

Figure 1b Placed on a prone board, good postural alignment and proper stability can be achieved with a belt across the hips. Rotation within the body axis and independent head movements are now made possible. Abnormal posture and tonus of the legs have been corrected. The closer the board is to the vertical position, the fewer demands are placed on righting head and trunk against gravity while lower extremity weight bearing increases.

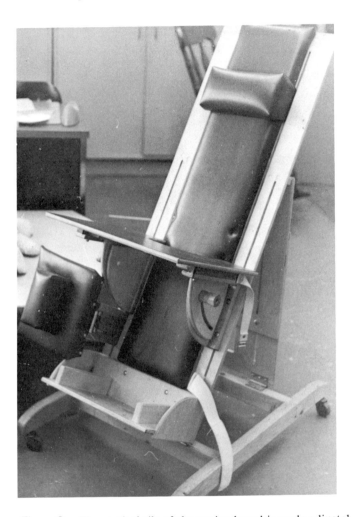

Figure 2a The vertical tilt of the supine board is made adjustable. A slight backward tilt encourages righting in the direction of flexion against gravity. A lap tray, adjustable in height and tilt, is used for security and for placement of toys. When indicated, a head support and a support across the thighs (not knees) can be attached.

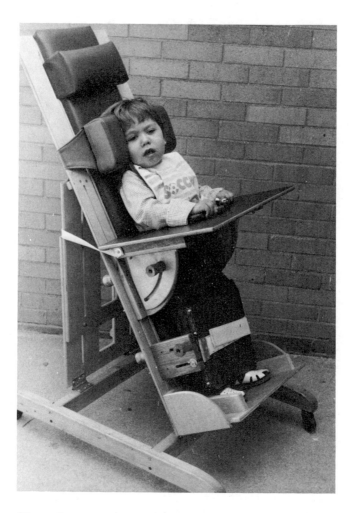

Figure 2b The supine board is used to facilitate the development of proper support tonus and righting against gravity in the vertical plane. A neutral posture of the pelvis allows proper hip extension and proper alignment of head in space.

Lateral trunk support corrects asymmetrical trunk posture. The chest cushion and lateral trunk supports should not be too high, but should allow the infant to move the arms freely for propping and play activities. Trunk support should not be so snug as to impede on the amplitude of ribcage motions for breathing.

The prone board facilitates extension against gravity while the supine board encourages the infant to counteract gravity by slightly flexing neck and upper trunk. The incline of the board determines the degree of antigravity activity which decreases progressively for upper trunk and head the closer the board is to the vertical position. As with all equipment, the prone and supine board should be used only for brief periods. The infant's position should be changed frequently. This is especially important for the severely disabled patient where the therapist has found one good position (after many attempts).

CARRYING

NORMAL DEVELOPMENT

During the first weeks of life a baby seems to struggle with balancing a relatively oversized head, succeeding only momentarily in attempts to hold the head upright while placed against a mother's supporting shoulder. In the second month, however, the infant can prevent severe head drops when being carried. By four months, good head righting and some trunk righting responses are established and parents report that the baby feels "firm and put together." The parent adjusts spontaneously by withdrawing total support of head and trunk.

ABNORMAL DEVELOPMENT

The infant with disturbed motor development requires prolonged postural support and is, therefore, held and carried in a more infantile, frequently reclined, position which gives little opportunity to right the head and trunk. The baby who is carried in a more upright position is often held with no regard to the shoulder girdle posture. Attempts to align head and shoulder girdle without a stable trunk posture result mostly in the head flopping from too much flexion to too much extension and elevation of the shoulder girdle. When lifting, parents tend to hold around the thorax and lift in a suspended supine position. The infant with motor difficulties is not able to align head and trunk (Fig. 3a). The head falls back or is pulled into extension.

The whole body may stiffen in response to the abnormal head posture which makes it very difficult to place the infant in a highchair or bathtub. The parent who carries the baby on the shoulder and always on the same side may reinforce an existing asymmetry of trunk and pelvis.

To cope with the numerous problems posed by poor head and trunk control, some parents place the infant into a baby carrier which is strapped around the parent's shoulders with the baby either in front or in back. The support provided by most baby carriers is not firm enough; the baby then sinks into too much flexion of the spine and consequently has to hyperextend the neck to lift the head. These infant carriers seem to be a poor imitation of an Indian custom where the baby is tightly wrapped in a long shawl which then is wrapped in many different ways around the mother's shoulders and trunk. The tight wrapping provides stability and maintains a close contact with the mother's body.

Handling. The infant experiences more normal righting and balancing when given proper support. It makes sense to take advantage of the fact that, during carrying, the parent's movements cause a continuous shift of the baby's center of gravity, therefore eliciting postural adjustments and readjustments. Principles for proper postural alignment are the same as those for seating and are therefore, only briefly outlined. A more upright position makes head and trunk righting easier. In addition to the orientation in space, the alignment between shoulder and pelvic girdle also determines the degree of extension or flexion of the spine (see "Positioning and Seating, Sitting Position"). Trunk balance is inhibited and the posture of the shoulder girdle impaired when the infant "hooks" one arm around mother's shoulder. Asymmetry of the pelvis leads to asymmetry of trunk and head.

1. The infant faces the parent, who places one arm across the infant's back and supports the pelvis and slightly flexed legs. The baby may sit on the parent's hipbone. Some trunk rotation and slight flexion of head and upper trunk is facilitated from the pelvis. Trunk support should be sufficient to make the infant feel secure but minimal enough to provide opportunity for normal balance reactions. Depending on the degree of head and trunk control, the infant turns head and trunk in response to the surroundings and in this position can respond to a variety of visual and auditory stimuli. Abnormal arm and should girdle postures, such as retraction, must be corrected.

2. The same upright position is maintained but the infant faces away from the parent (Fig. 3b). According to the degree of head and trunk control, the baby leans more or less against the parent's body. Both arms are brought

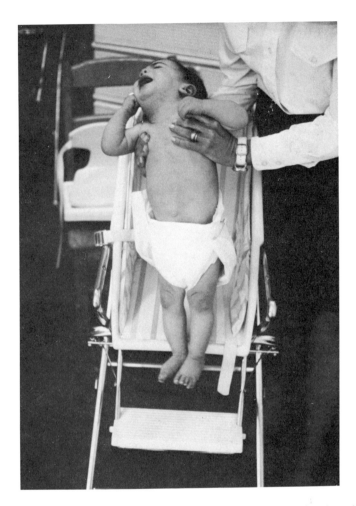

Figure 3a Hyperextension of head and neck may result when the infant is held in a suspended position while supported only around the thorax. The accompanying extensor hypertonicity makes it very difficult for the infant to sit in a highchair (from *The Infant with Cerebral Palsy: An Approach to Identification, Management and Treatment*, A. L. Scherzer. Private printing, New York, 1973).

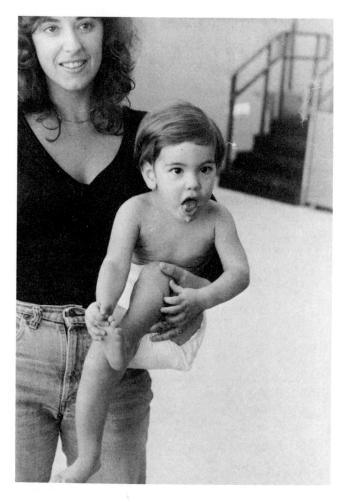

Figure 3b More appropriate head righting is facilitated when one or both hips are flexed while the infant is carried in an upright position. Pelvis and trunk need to be as upright as possible. Free observation of the surroundings and reaching can occur. Note the rotation within the body axis.

forward and confined between body and arm of the parent when retraction of the arms is a problem. The degree of hip extension is changeable as well as the extent to which the spine is extended or flexed, in the case of predominant extensor patterns, the trunk is slightly reclined. A component of trunk rotation can be introduced.

3. When it is not possible to correct abnormal retraction of arms with the above method, the parent is advised to hold the baby facing away while holding each leg, keeping the hips in flexion, pelvis and trunk upright. In this position, the parent's arms are then placed firmly against the baby's trunk, preventing shoulder retraction.

4. The arms can also be brought forward and over the parent's shoulder when the baby is held against the parent's shoulder and supported across the back.

5. Instead of always carrying the baby in an upright position, the parent may occasionally tilt the child onto the side to elicit dynamic lateral righting and amphibian reactions (Fig. 4). The infant is held around the arm on the lower (weight-bearing) side. This arm is brought into external rotation and complete abduction, which facilitates unilateral elongation of neck and trunk. The parent places the other arm between the infant's legs and holds the baby either around the trunk and chest or, if the infant displays a strong tendency toward shoulder retraction, around the other arm. When winging of the scapula is a problem, the parent can support the scapula on the elongated side instead of placing the hand on the infant's chest. The baby's head may rest on the abducted arm or on the parent's arm. When more support is needed, the infant's back rests against the parent's body. Postural adjustments can be varied by deviating from the horizontal plane or by tilting the infant partially toward supine or prone.

6. Complete prone position can be chosen for facilitation of extension against gravity. Again, the infant can be carried either in a completely horizontal or a more upright plane. The mother supports the infant under both externally rotated arms and places her other hand between the baby's legs to support the chest and abdomen from underneath.

Lifting. Difficulties of head righting are especially obvious when the infant is picked up from the supine position. Rather than lifting the baby in a suspended supine position, the parent is instructed to roll the baby partially toward one side which offers a better position for active flexion of neck and head. When lifting the infant out of the highchair or stroller, the parent

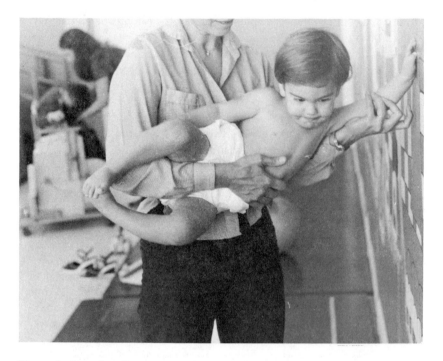

Figure 4 Occasionally, the infant may be tilted on his side when carried. Good posture of the shoulder girdle is achieved when the weight-bearing arm is supported in an externally rotated position. Lateral righting of head and trunk must be encouraged. (Photograph by Carol Herwig.)

places one arm across the baby's back, tilting the child's head and trunk slightly forward while supporting and holding both thighs with one or both hands.

BATHING

The difficulties of handling the developmentally impaired baby are enhanced during bathing because the baby's wet body becomes extremely slippery. The baby's and the parent's insecurity and tension may turn a basically joyful activity into one of apprehension.

Before placing the infant into the tub, the parent must carry and hold the baby in the most symmetrical and normal posture with the best possible alignment of head, trunk and pelvis. The tub should be equipped with a non-slip surface for better stability. When sufficient postural control cannot be provided by the parent, a commercially available bath seat is recommended, secured against sliding with suction cups or suspended from the rim of the tub. A child's swimming tub or a plastic clothes basket also provide some support and can be equipped with a seat belt if needed. Bathing in a small tub or in the kitchen sink makes it also easier for the mother to handle the infant who has poor postural control.

A floating toy or one tied to a string in front of the infant encourages proper head position and adds to the pleasure of taking a bath. It may be helpful to wrap the baby in a towel before being taken out of the tub.

DRESSING

NORMAL DEVELOPMENT
Toward the end of their first year, babies start to participate actively in undressing and dressing themselves. By that time they have learned that the arm goes through the sleeve: they hold out their feet to have shoes put on, or try to pull off their socks. By about 18 months to 2 years of age they can help in undressing but still need help in dressing for some time.

ABNORMAL DEVELOPMENT
The infant with CNS deficit shows considerable delay in dressing abilities. Some children may always need substantial help, but too often they are kept in a totally passive role. When sitting balance is impaired, the infant is usually dressed while lying flat on the back and cannot see and observe the parent while being dressed. Consequently, the child never learns how to participate.

Dressing Situation

Dressing is an activity where much learning can take place. Names of body parts and different clothing or actions, spatial relationships, laterality, crossing of midline, and sequencing of activities (socks before shoes) are some of the concepts which can be stressed during dressing. Balancing, weight shifting, and propping are motor reactions which occur naturally. Communication between the parent and the infant is an important aspect of this activity as of all activities of caretaking; the parent must be made aware of continuing the communication even though the infant may not be able to answer.

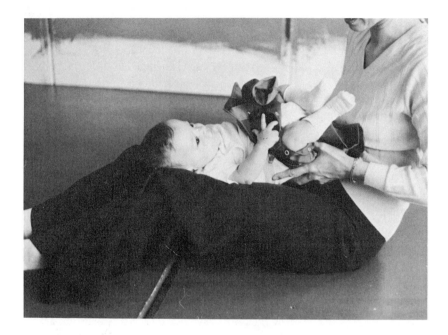

Figure 5 When the infant is dressed on the parent's lap, proper flexion of head and hips can be facilitated in the supine position. Correction of scapular retraction permits the infant to reach forward and participate in the activity. Rotation within the body axis and lateral weight shifting can easily be incorporated. (Photograph by Marion Madigan.)

Positions for Dressing

SUPINE
Flexion against gravity can be facilitated when the infant is dressed in the supine position. The legs are elevated which makes it possible for the infant to watch how pants, socks, and shoes are put on or taken off. With some encouragement the baby may reach toward the feet and help more or less with the chore. A weight shift to one side can be easily incorporated and stressed during this activity and may lead to rolling. Rolling the baby from side to side is necessary when the shirt is to be put on in this position. Dressing in supine can be carried out on the dressing table but also very comfortably on the parent's lap (Fig. 5).

SITTING

The infant who has achieved some trunk control is seated on the dressing table and dressed from the front. This is an excellent time to practice and improve sitting balance, because the center of gravity is continuously shifted. Propping on the hands is encouraged initially while the parent lifts the baby's foot and leg to put on socks, shoes, and pants. Later, the baby may be able to balance while pushing the limbs or head through garment openings. Gradually, the infant participates more in the activity, for example, pulling off a sock after the parent has pulled it halfway down over the heel. The baby who cannot participate on this level is guided from shoulder or arm.

The infant who is less independent in sitting is dressed with the parent providing support from behind. Sitting on the parent's lap during dressing allows even more control of trunk and arm movements. In addition, weight shifting can be accentuated when the mother moves her legs. Trunk rotation and guidance from shoulder or arm are used to facilitate reaching (Fig. 6).

SIDE LYING

In the side-lying position the baby is also able to observe dressing activities. The infant who is hypertonic while lying face upward may be reasonably relaxed when turned side ways and thus may be able to stretch arms forward to reach garments and touch legs. To encourage lateral righting and proper head position, the head should be supported on a small pillow or folded towel.

PRONE

Dressing in prone is especially suited for babies with a strong tendency to push into extension. It is best carried out with the infant lying on the parent's lap, where sweaters and shirts can easily be pulled off in a backward to forward motion. This facilitates flexion of the neck while removing a garment front to backward over the head may reinforce extension. Lateral weight shift and trunk rotation can be practiced during dressing. The parent should be instructed to support the infant well under the stomach if the infant has a tendency to sway back. Caution is also indicated when the infant tends to pull into flexion from the arms. Instead of having the arms hang over the parent's leg they should be brought forward into full overhead flexion and some external rotation while weight bearing occurs on the long side of the arms. This position cannot be used to encourage self-dressing, but can be beneficial for the parent of a stiff baby.

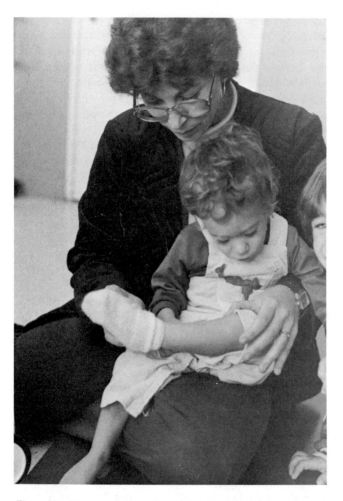

Figure 6 Sitting balance is provided with support from behind. The posture of the left leg decreases extensor spasticity and reinforces more dissociated leg movements. When seated upright and securely supported, the infant can observe and participate in undressing and dressing.

Handling Principles

Parents need advice on specific handling principles to improve and facilitate dressing. Care should be taken not to elicit a stretch reflex by pulling on the infant's hand while trying to get an arm through a sleeve. An increase of flexor tonus may be the response to this pull and hamper cooperation. It is much easier to straighten the arm by pushing the elbow forward and upward. The parent of a hemiplegic or very asymmetrically impaired infant is advised to put the garments on the more affected limbs first. Specific handling techniques are also required for putting on shoes when the infant plantarflexes the ankles tightly and curls the toes. These difficulties are reduced when the leg is brought into flexion and foot and toes are dorsiflexed while the heel is loaded for weight bearing. Unlacing and opening the shoes completely makes it possible to control and correct the position of foot and toes in the shoe. Once the toes are dorsiflexed they can be held in this position by pulling back on the infant's sock near the toes. If the infant pulls the heel up, the parent provides downward pressure from the flexed knee before lacing the shoe.

Clothes

The right choice of clothes plays some part in reducing the difficulties in dressing. To put on a tight turtleneck or overall outfit may require extensive stretching and twisting of the limbs and can leave both the infant and the parent frustrated. It is much easier to pull arms through garments with the opening and fastenings in the back. Large openings and clothes that can be stretched reduce the necessity for moving limbs in complicated and difficult patterns. However, foot coverings of elastic material can reinforce clawing of the toes and should not be pulled too tight.

MOBILITY

During the second half of the first year a baby develops different and increasingly more effective forms of locomotion. The infant with CNS impairment, on the other hand, is very restricted in mode of progression and may use excessive extensor patterns while pushing along in supine, or excessive flexor tonus may result from pulling forward in prone. The reinforcement of asymmetrical postures is also a concern during locomotion. The most severely impaired infant may experience considerable frustration at not being able to move around without assistance.

It is no surprise then that both infant and parent are delighted to find
that a baby walker provides this mobility. As discussed earlier in this chapter
("Standing with Support"), the disadvantages in most cases outweigh the advantages of such a walker. Other means of providing mobility should be
found.

Equipment

Scooter boards are in wide use. Considering how strenuous the prone position
is, they are of little use for the severely affected child. Without sufficient
postural control, the effort involved increases hypertonicity and makes it
even more difficult for the infant to maneuver the equipment. The toddler
is better served using mobility equipment in supported sitting, such as different
types of "toddler riders" and, later on, tricycles. They require a thoughtful
design. Pelvis and trunk must be stabilized in an upright position to allow for
the necessary mobility of the limbs. Applicable concepts have been discussed
in Positioning and Seating. When internal rotation and adduction of the hips
need modification, a wedge is placed between both thighs. Scapular protraction and internal rotation of the shoulders can be neutralized when the
handlebars are changed from horizontal to vertical position.

FEEDING

Difficulties in feeding the infant with CNS deficit may seriously interfere
with a family's daily routine. Impaired oral development often results in unacceptably long feeding sessions, and can cause considerable frustration and
anxiety for infant and parent.

Immediate intervention is necessary to interrupt and reduce these adverse
influences and is of primary concern where malnutrition is a possibility.
Appropriate feeding management helps to counteract the development of abnormal and possibly grotesque feeding patterns which may keep patients
dependent for the rest of their lives, limiting social integration and acceptance. The specific information obtained during the oral evaluation and the
recommendations emerging from this assessment constitute the basis of a
feeding program. This program has to consider all factors influencing abnormal oral behavior.

Positioning

Posture and position accompanying feeding should be considered first.
Alignment and stability of head, neck and upper trunk greatly influences

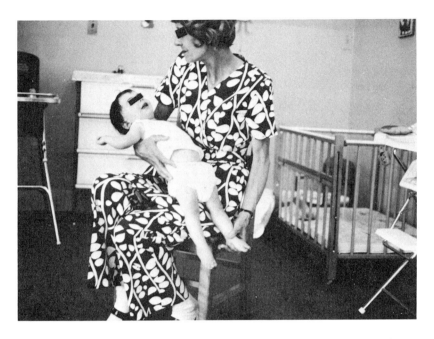

Figure 7a Extensor spasticity is aggravated in this poorly supported supine position. Head and arms are pulled back and the back arches, which makes it very difficult to achieve any oral control. In addition, this position severely limits the infant's active interaction with the environment. (From *The Infant with Cerebral Palsy: An Approach to Identification, Management and Treatment*. A. L. Scherzer. Private printing, New York, 1973.)

oral posture and function. Infants are often fed in a reclined position when sitting balance is impaired and when food cannot be transferred back by the tongue (Fig. 7a). A child kept in this disadvantageous posture cannot develop active manipulation of the food and will always rely on the assistance of gravity for swallowing. It is therefore imperative to select a position as upright and symmetrical as possible. Providing sufficient postural support and good stability makes the task easier for everyone involved. Improving the infant's

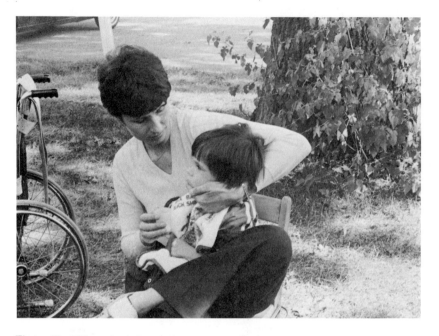

Figure 7b When the infant is fed seated on the parent's lap it is important to stress an upright posture of head and trunk. Support to the low and mid-back may be required to achieve an upright head posture. The parent's knee can be used to support the child's back. "Jaw control" also corrects any tendency to head retraction or turning and tilting of the head. The arms are brought forward for proper posture of the shoulder girdle. The grasp around the jaw monitors oral posture and movement (see text).

position may result in spontaneous improvement of vegetative functions. Optimal feeding patterns seem to be linked to optimal positioning in the patient with CNS deficit.

By 5 to 6 months of age the normal baby has developed sufficient sitting balance to be fed while sitting in the highchair. When possible, the developmentally impaired infant should also be fed sitting in a highchair or seat insert. Guidelines for the design of corrective and supportive seating arrangements have been discussed previously (see "Positioning and Seating, Sitting Position").

The same concepts for postural control apply to the infant who is fed on the parent's lap (Fig. 7b). Placing one foot on a stool helps the parent to increase the amount of the infant's hip flexion, or, with the other leg, to support the baby's back against the knee, while resting the arm on the knee or on a nearby table. It is important that the seating arrangement be comfortable for the infant and the parent otherwise it will deteriorate during the feeding session.

Another feeding position has been described by Helen Mueller. She places the infant with poor head control on a wedge or pillow in a semireclined position. Sufficient flexion of the head and hips counteracts abnormal extensor patterns. For this arrangement, the infant sits on the parent's lap facing the parent, a wedge or pillow is placed behind the child's head and back while leaning against the edge of a table.

James Bosma recommends feeding the child with swallowing problems in prone. Proper positioning in prone and on the prone board has been described previously (see "Standing with Support"). It should again be stressed that sufficient extension against gravity is necessary for adequate head control in prone. The severely hypotonic infant may raise the head with excessive extensor tonus or may rest too heavily on the chin when given "jaw control" (see "Jaw Control"). This can lead to abnormally high tonus in the oral area. Positioning on the prone board in a more upright position diminishes these problems.

Attention also should be given to the parent's position in relation to the infant. Placement of the food and how the parent approaches the infant also influence head position. For example, presenting the food from above encourages too much head extension. To correct hyperextension of the neck and reinforce midline orientation the food should be presented from the front.

Jaw Control

Although appropriate positioning greatly improves oral function, further control of oral responses may be indicated for the severely impaired patient. This specific control can be achieved with a facial grasp or "jaw control." By gently cupping the chin, the head can be moved on the spine in a backward, upward motion. This lowers the chin while elongating the neck and sliding the head back. After establishing alignment and stability of head and neck, movements of jaw, lips and tongue will be better graded and, if necessary, can be guided with input to mandible, lower lip, or cheeks. Input should never be strong enough to elicit resistance. Instead, the therapist waits for the infant to adapt as far as feels comfortable, which will be short of a perfect posture. Some infants may need help with stability of the upper trunk which can be done from the ribcage. To correct sinking or pulling into flexion, the direction of this input should be away from midline upward and backward, as if to stabilize the ribs onto the spine. It must be very gentle to avoid impinging on respiration. To correct too much extension, a very gentle input is directed from the upper ribcage back into the low thoracic spine.

The facial grasp can be applied from the side and from the front (see Fig. 7b). The parent will need some practice and occasional supervision by the therapist to become efficient in these techniques. Common errors are to pull the chin too far forward, which results in hyperextension of the neck, to pull the mandible to one side, or to turn the head laterally. As the infant gains more control over the oral mechanism, the use of the facial grasp is no longer required and should be gradually discontinued. After establishing sufficient control of posture and oral responses the infant is prepared for food intake.

Feeding Procedures

To facilitate normal feeding patterns and inhibit abnormal feeding responses, the therapist must have a thorough knowledge of oral development. Both normal and abnormal feeding patterns as well as underlying components and subskills have been described in the section of feeding evaluation (see Chap. 5).

Sucking. Sucking at the breast is easier for the infant with CNS impairment if held in a more upright position or when placed on one side. Extensor patterns should be corrected, especially retraction of shoulders, arms, and head. Some support under the chin (jaw control) may improve the efficiency of the suck-swallow pattern.

The success of bottle drinking depends in great part on the proper selection of the nipple. A nipple that is too long for the infant's mouth hinders proper tongue movements. A nipple with a big opening allows free and constant flowing of the liquid into the mouth, which the infant will not be able to regulate through the sucking action. The abundance of liquid is a particular problem for the infant with swallowing difficulties. The therapist, therefore, should personally test the nipple by tilting the bottle upside down.

There should be no free and constant flow of liquid. A short round nipple with a small opening is the proper choice. The use of a "bottle straw" which can be attached to any nipple allows the infant to empty the bottle without tilting the head back and is very conducive to feeding the handicapped infant. The consistency, taste, and temperature of the liquid chosen may also influence sucking patterns. Responses to different qualities of liquids are described below.

Cup drinking. The normal infant initiates cup drinking by the age of 5 to 6 months. The infant with feeding difficulties is usually fed by bottle for a much longer time. When cup drinking is finally initiated, the baby is frequently given a spouted cup which encourages the child to retain primitive or abnormal sucking patterns. The handicapped infant is thus not given a fair chance to develop more mature feeding habits. The exaggerated licking action of the tongue and lack of lip movements yield very inefficient drinking patterns, especially for cup drinking. Early initiation of cup drinking under proper guidance helps to counteract the habituation of poor feeding patterns and is an important step in fostering more normal development.

The facial grasp procedure helps to reduce a predominant suck by stabilizing the jaw, decreasing lingual and mandibular movements, and facilitating discrete lip movements. Furthermore, sipping movements are stimulated by the sensory input of the liquid touching the lips. This means that the cup should not be placed too far into the mouth. Placing the cup on the teeth or biting surface does not encourage sipping, but reinforces sucking and biting. Remember that the aim is to have the infant take the liquid in with the lips and not the tongue. Jaw and lip closure must also be facilitated during swallowing.

It is particularly difficult for the handicapped baby to manipulate thin and watery liquids. Slightly thickened liquids provide a stronger stimulus for labial sipping movements and are easier to gather into a bolus for swallowing. Creamed soups, melted ice cream, nectars, loose puddings, and milk shakes are good choices. Gradually, liquids of thinner consistency are included in the diet. Taste and temperature should be considered. Sweet substances reinforce sucking. Taste can also affect the flow of saliva; some fruits, flavors such as apple, lemon, and orange stimulate increased salivation, as does chocolate. These liquids should not be given to infants with severe swallowing difficulties. Extreme temperatures often elicit hypertonicity in the oral area.

Another consideration is size and composition of the cup. A small cup can be emptied more easily than a large one, without having to tilt the head too far back. The cup should be made of a pliable, durable material, especially for the infant with an obligatory bite reflex. Breakable plastic cups must be avoided. The pliability of a cup allows the parent to form a spout to reduce spilling when the infant cannot yet sip efficiently. Helen Mueller suggests cutting a notch out of the rim to allow room for the nose and make it possible to empty the cup without tilting the head too far back. It also helps the parent to monitor the flow of liquid.

Spoon feeding. Many mothers introduce one or two spoonfuls of solids by the time the baby is about 3 months old, which is shortly after the infant learns to swallow voluntarily. Solids form a substantial part of the diet of a 5- or 6-month-old baby. The switch from sucking to effective handling of solids is, of course, gradual. Initial attempts at spoonfeeding are not very successful because the infant uses sucking motions. Spoonfeeding the infant who has not only primitive feeding reflexes but also abnormal sucking and abnormal swallowing patterns is therefore a greater challenge.

In order to monitor abnormal sucking and swallowing patterns, jaw control is essential. Better postural and mandibular stability decrease exaggerated opening of the mouth which is one component of an abnormal suck. Jaw stability also modifies and weakens exaggerated tongue motions and an obligatory suck. To further inhibit the forward thrusting of the tongue, downward pressure on the tongue can be applied with the spoon. This accentuated sensory input may also prompt proper action of the lips for taking the food off the spoon. The spoon should not be put too far into the mouth and should be removed quickly before the baby bites down on it. It should always be held horizontally. Care must be taken not to tilt the spoon nor scrape it along the teeth since this may result in retraction of the lips. Assistance for jaw and lip closure is to be continued until swallowing has occurred. The upper lip should not be pulled down passively because the hypersensitive infant reacts to this with spasticity. Lip closure and protrusion of the lips are elicited more successfully from the lower lip or the cheeks.

Proper selection of the food contributes to the success of spoon feeding. As with cup drinking, thinner consistencies are difficult to control and aggravate drooling. Mixed consistencies, such as vegetable soups and some prepared baby food dinners should not be presented to the infant with impaired oral perception and disturbed coordination. It requires special skill to sort and manipulate different consistencies. Foods such as mashed potatoes, cooked cereals, or puddings are recommended for initial attempts at spoonfeeding. Most foods can be prepared in the baby strainer without liquifying them. Increasing the repertoire of textures, tastes, and temperatures is a long-term goal of this program.

Shape, size, and material of the spoon must be taken into account. For safety reasons, breakable plastic utensils should be excluded. Teflon-coated or rubber tipped spoons are helpful for infants with a strong bite response. The depth of the spoon's bowl affects lip activity and must be adjusted to the infant's capabilities. A flat metal spoon, such as the "mother care" spoon makes removal of the food easier. A spoon with a very small, narrow bowl which can be placed on the tongue without hitting the lingual sides of the teeth is effective for feeding the infant with a strong bite reflex.

Biting and chewing. As a first step in teaching the patient how to manipulate solids, he or she must be assisted in the inhibition of the suck and bite reflexes. Jaw control suppresses extreme depression of the mandible and allows chewing or munching movements. The jaw should not be moved passively in a rotary motion so as not to interfere with the coordination between movements of lips, tongue, and jaw. Introducing the food from the side and placing it directly on the chewing surface discourages sucking and facilitates tongue lateralization. It may be necessary initially not only to place the food on the biting surface but also to hold it there during the infant's attempts at chewing. This will influence the selection of food.

As with drinking and spoonfeeding, the type of food presented to the infant can drastically affect success or failure. Baby foods, sandwiches, and peanut butter and jelly encourage sucking. Crackers are too dry and tend to scatter, making it difficult to form a bolus. Crusts and hard bread, dried fruits, hard cheese, cooked vegetables, and strips of meat are recommended textures. Taste and temperature again must be considered.

The nutritional value of food is especially important for the infant with severe feeding problems and the advice of a dietician is strongly recommended. Frequent and short feeding sessions may work best when feeding problems are serious.

Self-feeding. Infants begin to fingerfeed at 5 to 6 months of age and handle utensils with moderate spilling by about 2 years of age. The handicapped child may never achieve total independence, but should nevertheless, be encouraged to participate as actively as possible. Otherwise, total dependence on others for feeding can pose emotional and social problems later. Appropriate support, assistance, and specific adaptations may be required.

An infant can only fingerfeed or handle utensils when seated securely without the need of hands for support. Guidelines for seating have been given in the preceding section.

The selection of food should follow the above recommendations.

When utensils are used, their safety has to be considered. Breakable plastic should not be used. The infant who tightly fists hands when grasping should be given a spoon with a built-up handle in order to widen the grasp. The parent may teach self-feeding effectively by stabilizing the spoon with thumb against the infant's palm. The parent's fingers at the dorsum of the infant's hand guide the infant's hand movements. Taking the food off the plate may be as challenging as bringing the food into the mouth. The food is easily pushed off the plate or the plate slides away. A plate with a high curved rim is very helpful and can be further stabilized by being placed on a nonskid pad.

The hand not being used for feeding should be placed on the table to diminish associated reactions and ensure trunk symmetry. This is especially important for the hemiplegic child.

It is important not to overlook oral reactions when teaching the infant how to manipulate different feeding utensils. The effort used in self-feeding can elicit abnormal oral tonus and associated reactions in the oral area. To reduce this abnormal sensory feedback, it is recommended that the infant's hand be guided and jaw control is provided until independence in the most normal fashion is achieved.

ORAL HYGIENE

Oral hygiene is of special importance in the infant with feeding problems, since the restricted diet and lack of intrinsic tongue movements do not help to clean teeth, gums, and palate. Without proper oral care, gums deteriorate, especially in the infant who is on anticonvulsive medication.

Even before teeth erupt, the gums should be cleaned after each feeding with a moist towel wrapped around the parent's finger or a toothbrush with a soft cylindrical head, such as the NUK toothbrush trainer. This can also be used for oral stimulation, adapted to the baby's level of tolerance, while controlling motor responses with proper techniques of jaw control. In the hypersensitive infant, very light touch elicits very strong reactions, and the parent should be careful not to elicit a gag reflex.

Later on, a small, soft toothbrush is introduced and rinsing of the mouth is carried out with warm water. To facilitate spitting, head flexion is important and the infant can be further assisted with gentle forward pressure toward the cheeks.

This feeding program, it is hoped, will enable the infant to properly manage a healthy diet and is conducive to dental and oral health.

SUMMARY

The infant with sensorimotor deficit is often handled in a way that encourages primitive and passive behavior. When the parent adjusts to the infant's abnormal postural reactions, abnormal postures and movements are established and become habitual. Reinforcement of primitive and abnormal behavior aggravates developmental delay.

Intervention in the form of specific handling methods has been described in this chapter and is designed to interrupt abnormal sensorimotor behavior while fostering more normal development. The handicapped infant is able to participate in dressing and feeding activities actively when placed in more advantageous positions and provided with corrective, proximal support. When well-positioned and securely seated, the child can manipulate and investigate toys. For the severely impaired infant, play is made possible with electronic toys. A wide variety of electronic switches can be adapted to regular toys. With appropriate guidance, the parent gains skill and confidence in handling the infant who lacks adequate postural control. The parent also learns to foster the infant's independence.

To optimize the patient's potential and encourage the development of mature patterns of posture and movement it is necessary to provide more specific handling and more selective stimulation through a well-designed treatment program.

APPENDIX Infant Management Evaluation

Name:	Birth date:	Chart no.:
Diagnosis:	Date:	Examiner:

   I.   General Impressions (family situation, daily routine, activities and habits, availability and appropriateness of toys):

  II.   Functional Abilities and Areas of Strength (head control, trunk control, manipulative skills, ability to adjust to handling, awareness, social/physical interaction, grasp patterns, eye-hand coordination):

 III.   Areas of Major Difficulties:

 IV.   Carrying, Lifting:
1.   Present procedures (postural adaptations, active participation by infant, approach by parent, tolerance towards handling):

2.   Postural Reactions Interfering with Proper Adaptations to Being Carried:

poor head control	_____	pronounced flexion of lumbar
poor trunk and shoulder girdle		spine _____
stability	_____	one/both arms retracted _____
asymmetry (head,		excessive, uncontrolled
spine, pelvis)	_____	movements _____
poor tolerance toward		others:
handling	_____	

3.   Risk for Development of Contractures, Deformities:

4.   Postural Corrections and Support Needed for Optimal Function:

hip flexion	_____	trunk rotation _____
back support (lumbar)	_____	hands to midline _____
trunk vertical, pelvis		extended posture (prone) _____
level	_____	others:
hips abducted	_____	

5.   Summary:

6.   Recommendations:

V. Positioning:
1. Present Procedures

2. Evaluation of Postural Adaptations and Functional Abilities:
   Supine
a. Spontaneous Postures, Motor Functions:

b. Postural Corrections and Support Provided Yielding Functional Abilities:

head flexed	flexed legs supported	shoulder support		
_____	_____	_____	hands to midline, symmetry	_____
_____	_____	_____	goal directed reach, play	_____
_____	_____	_____	changes position	_____
_____	_____	_____	equilibrium reactions	_____

Prone
a. Spontaneous Postures, Motor Functions:

b. Postural Corrections and Support Provided Yielding Functional Abilities:

hips extended	pelvis stabilized	on incline		
_____	_____	_____	free head movements, neck elongated	_____
_____	_____	_____	leans on elbows	_____
_____	_____	_____	hands	_____
_____	_____	_____	reaches for toys	_____
_____	_____	_____	changes position	_____
_____	_____	_____	equilibrium reactions	_____

Sidelying
a. Spontaneous Postures, Motor Functions:

b. Postural Corrections and Support Provided Yielding Functional Abilities:

head elevated	trunk supported (back)	(front)		
_____	_____	_____	hands to midline, plays	_____
_____	_____	_____	changes position	_____
_____			equilibrium reactions	_____

Sitting: on floor; in highchair, chair; on parent's lap
a. Spontaneous Postures, Motor Functions:

b. Postural Corrections and Support Provided Yielding Functional Abilities

hip flexion 90°	lumbar spine supported	back vertical	back reclined	knees flexed		
___	___	___	___	___	symmetry (head, trunk, pelvis)	___
___	___	___	___	___	head control, neck	
___	___	___	___	___	elongation	___
___	___	___	___	___	leans on hands	___
___	___	___	___	___	hands free for play	___
___	___	___	___	___	equilibrium reactions	___
___	___	___	___	___	changes positions	___

3. Summary:

4. Recommendations:
Positioning, Postural Alignment:

Equipment:

Adaptations to highchair, stroller, mobility equipment:

VI. Dressing
1. Present Procedures (postural adaptations and active participation by infant, approach by parent, type of clothing):

2. Postural Reactions Interfering with Dressing:

poor sitting balance	___	excessive uncontrolled
thrust into extension	___	movements ___
pull into flexion	___	tight flexion of arms, fisted
	___	hands ___
tight adduction of hips	___	others ___
plantar flexed ankles, curled toes	___	

3. Positioning and Handling Procedures for Optimal Function:

Supine:	legs flexed	_____	incorporating trunk rotation _____
	flexion of head	_____	pushing arms through sleeves
Sitting:	trunk support	_____	(no pull) _____
	hip flexion	_____	flexing hips, knees _____
Prone		_____	ankles, toes dorsiflexed _____
Sidelying		_____	others _____

4. Summary:

5. Recommendations:
Positioning:

Handling:

Clothes:

VII. Feeding
1. Present Procedures:
Positioning (infant's posture, approach by parent, equipment):

Oral posture, tonus, movements (jaws, lips, tongue):

at rest:

during sucking:

during spoon feeding:

during biting, chewing:

during self-feeding:

2. Factors Interfering with Food Intake:

Posture:

Approach by parent:

Selection of food, utensils:

Abnormal oral tonus, abnormal oral sensitivity:

Primitive/abnormal oral reflexes:
rooting _____suck–swallow _____ phasic bite _____
tonic bite _____ hyperactive gag _____ hypoactive gag _____

Structural deformities:

Teething:

Respiratory problems:

Choking, vomiting:

3. Intervention and Its Effect on Feeding:

Positioning:
   upright position of head, trunk:

   head slightly flexed:

   support to lumbar spine:

   prone position:

   sidelying:

Selection of food as to consistency, taste, temperature, texture:

Selection of utensils:
   nipple size, size of opening:

   rigid straw:

   size and shape of cup:

   size and shape of spoon:

Handling:
   jaw control:

   approach from front:

spoon held horizontally:

food placed on biting surface:

guidance for self-feeding:

4. Summary:

5. Recommendations:

Positioning:

Handling:

Food, Utensils:

VIII. Bathing
1. Present Procedures (postural adaptations, active participation by infant, approach by parent, equipment):

2. Postural Reactions Interfering with Bathing:

poor head control	_____	hypotonic ("frog") posture	_____
poor trunk control	_____	excessive, uncontrolled	
thrust into extension	_____	movements	_____
pronounced flexion	_____	others:	

3. Postural Corrections and Support Needed for Optimal Function:

head supported in flexion	_____	midline orientation, symmetry	_____
hips flexed	_____		
trunk supported	_____	others:	

4. Summary:

5. Recommendations:

Positioning:

Handling:

Equipment:

IX. Postural Tonus
     normal _____ hypotonic _____ hypertonic _____ rigid _____
     fluctuating _____
     Change of tonus with stimulation, handling, movement:

X.   Sensitivity (kinesthetic, tactile, auditory, visual stimuli):

XI. Factors Interfering with Daily Care
hypertonicity extensor   ____   poor head control, poor righting ____
hypertonicity flexor   ____   poor balance and proximal
lack of support tonus   ____   stability   ____
postural asymmetry   ____   hypersensitivity toward
lack of mobility   ____   handling   ____
                                         unresponsiveness   ____
                                         others:

XII. Risk for Developing Contractures, Deformities:

XIII. Additional Remarks:

XIV. Summary

Displayed behavior seems to be typical _____, if not give apparent reason:

BIBLIOGRAPHY

Ardran, G. M., Kemp, F. H., and Lind, J. A cineradiographic study of bottle feeding, *Br. J. Radiol.* 31:11, 1958.

Ardran, G. M., Kemp, F. H., and Lind, J. A cineradiographic study of breast feeding. *Br. J. Radiol.* 31:154, 1958.

Ardran, G. M., and Kemp, F. H. Some important factors in the assessment of oro-pharyngeal function. *Dev. Med. Child Neurol.* 12:158-166, 1970.

Bobath, B. The very early treatment of cerebral palsy. *Dev. Med. Child Neurol.* 9:373-390, 1967.

Bosma, J. F. Human infant oral function. In Bosma, J. (Ed.), Symposium on Oral Sensation and Perception. Springfield, IL., Charles C Thomas, pp. 98-111, 1967.

Bosma, J. F. Physiology of the mouth, pharynx and esophagus. In Otolaryngology. Philadelphia, Saunders, 1973, pp. 356-370.

Bosma, J. F. (Ed.). Fourth Symposium on Oral Sensation and Perception. Washington, D.C., U.S. Government Printing Office, 1973.

Bosma, J. F., and Showacre, J. (Eds.). Development of Upper Respiratory Anatomy and Function (Symposium). Washington, D.C., U.S. Government Printing Office, 1975.

Davis, L. F. Pre-speech. In Connor, P., Williamson, G., and Siep, J. (Eds.), Program Guide for Infants and Toddlers with Neuromotor and Other Developmental Disabilities. New York, Teachers College Press, 1979, pp. 183-205.

Doty, R. W., and Bosma, J. F. An electromyographic analysis of reflex deglutition. *J. Neurophysiol.* 19:44-60, 1956.

Finnie, N. R. Handling the Young Cerebral Palsied Child at Home (2nd ed). New York, Dutton, 1975.

Hochleitner, M. Betreuung des cerebral bewegungsgestörten Säuglings (Handling), Mutteranleitung. Göttingen, Institut für den Wissenschaftlichen Film, Medizin 4, 12, C 1241, 1978.

Illingworth, R. S. Sucking and swallowing difficulties in infancy: diagnostic problems of dysphagia. *Arch. Dis. Child.* 44:238, 1969.

Ingram, T. T. S. Clinical significance of the infantile feeding reflexes. *Dev. Med. Child Neurol.* 4:159-169, 1962.

Nelson, Ch. Self-Feeding Patterns. In Selected Proceedings from Barbro Salek Memorial Symposium. NDTA, Oak Park, IL, 1984.

Morris, S. E. Pre-Feeding Skills. Therapy Skill Builders, Tucson, AZ, 1987.

Morris, S. E. Program Guidelines for Children with Feeding Problems. Edison, N.J., Childcraft Educational Corp., 1977.

Mueller, H. A. Facilitating feeding and pre-speech. In Pearons, P. H., and Williams, C. E. (Eds), Physical Therapy Services in the Developmental Disabilities. Springfield, IL, Charles C Thomas, 1972, pp. 283-310.

Mueller, H. A. Feeding. In Finnie, N. (Ed.), Handling the Young Cerebral Palsied Child at Home, New York, Dutton, 1975.

Sameroff, A. J. Reflexive and operant aspects of sucking behavior in early infancy. In Bosma, J. F. (Ed.), Fourth Symposium on Oral Sensation and Perception. Washington, D.C., U.S. Government Printing Office, 1973, pp. 135-151.

Staller, J. An approach to adaptive seating. In Selected Proceedings from Barbro Salek Memorial Symposium. NDTA, Oak Park, IL, 1984.

Straub, J. Malfunction of the tongue: Abnormal swallowing, its cause, effects and results in relation to orthodontic treatment and speech therapy. *Am. J. Orthodon*. 46:404-424, 1960.

Wilder, C. N. Respiratory Patterns. In Infants: Birth to Eight Months of Age. Unpublished doctoral dissertation. New York, Teachers College, Columbia University, 1972.

Willoughby, M., Tscharnuter, I., and Fabricant, P. Treatment Approaches to the Oral Developmental Needs in Cerebral Palsy. Instructional course lecture, American Academy for Cerebral Palsy, 1974, 1975, 1976.

Wilson, J. M. Physical Therapy and infant home management programs. Proceedings from the Comprehensive Management of Infants at Risk for CNS Deficit, May 1974. Chapel Hill, Division of Physical Therapy, University of North Carolina, Chapel Hill, 1975.

Wilson, J. M. (Ed.). Oral Motor Function and Dysfunction in Children. Proceedings, May 1977. Chapel Hill, N.C., Division of Physical Therapy, University of North Carolina, Chapel Hill, 1978.

8

Treatment

Treatment of the infant with symptoms of cerebral palsy and related sensorimotor deficits must include the family. Family involvement in handling the
infant should go beyond intervention methods of home management discussed in Chapter 7 to include treatment procedures. When the parent carries
out a home therapy program, the infant is guided and assisted in development on a daily basis and within a daily routine.

The therapist must nevertheless help the parent to put the home management and therapy program into the right perspective so as not to disturb the
parent-child relationship. Focusing the attention exclusively on the infant's
disabilities hampers rather than fosters overall development. Abnormal
motor patterns can be overemphasized. It is only the continuous repetition
of these patterns which interferes with normal development. The parent—and
the therapist—must understand that there are moments where therapeutic
intervention must be secondary.

Instructions given to the parent must be thorough and detailed enough to
assure the quality of the home program. Handling techniques must be adapted to the skills of the parent and may consequently differ from the techniques the therapist applies to the same activity.

Good parent training ensures not only an intensive, continuous treatment
program for the infant but frees the therapist to serve more patients. In accordance with this concept the therapist's role is not only to administer a
treatment remedy but also, to a great extent, to act as advisor for the family.

NEURODEVELOPMENTAL APPROACH

Coordination of Movement Patterns

A major concept of this treatment approach is based on the conclusion that a lesion of the central nervous system (CNS) results in a loss of movement and not in a paresis of muscles [1]. Furthermore, it is believed that new motor skills are learned by learning "movement patterns and not a sequence of a mosaic of activation of specific muscles" [2]. Stretching and strengthening of individual muscles are consequently not considered to be therapeutic. Instead, a much broader approach must be chosen. In learning new motor skills, the focus is mainly on the coordination of movement patterns and their accompanying postures.

Relation Between Movement, Posture, and Postural Tonus

Normal movement patterns are accompanied by postures which are changing and therefore dynamic [3]. Postures also precede and facilitate movement (some of these postures have been described in Chap. 4). The infant with a restricted repertoire of postures is limited in purposeful movements.

Efficient postures and movements require normal strength, adaptibility and distribution of postural tonus. In therapy, the close interplay between movement, posture, and tonus is utilized. Modification of any one of these funtions changes the others. For example, tonus can be changed by correcting abnormal postural alignment which, in turn, makes possible more normal movement patterns.

Automatic and Voluntary Movements

Another concept implies that proper adaptation of posture and tonus, and maintenance of balance are normally regulated by subcortical centers. Postural adaptations are mostly automatic, freeing higher cortical centers for planning intentional motor acts and a variety of mental and learning processes.

Patterns of voluntary movements are based on automatic postural reactions, such as righting, equilibrium, and other protective reactions [4] as well as on primary motor patterns which emerge in utero [5].

The goal of therapy is to elicit appropriate automatic reactions in response to handling. Working on an automatic level has the additional advantage of diminishing the increasing hypertonicity often resulting from the effort and anticipation involved in a remeditated act. The fact that motor responses can be elicited on an automatic level makes this approach largely independent of the patient's level of mental function and cooperation. Its application is therefore well-suited to the young infant.

Active Participation

The learning of new motor skills requires that they be carried out actively. It is not sufficient to maneuver the infant through different motor patterns while passive. An activity can be active even when assistance and support are provided, but this assistance must be kept at an optimal level to ensure active participation of the infant without eliciting an abnormal response as a result of stress and effort.

Automatic motor responses, such as righting and equilibrium reactions, although elicited on a subconscious level are as active as voluntary motions.

Interplay Between Various Motor Patterns

In normal development, primary motor patterns as primitive reflexes and early righting reactions, become increasingly complex or fade out as more mature automatic responses, such as equilibrium reactions emerge. In cerebral palsy, primitive patterns become increasingly more inefficient and abnormal, leading to secondary compensations. Although secondary compensations may be more obvious, underlying primary problems must be addressed.

Persistence of poorly integrated motor patterns form a poor neurological as well as biomechanical base for the development of more complex motor skills.

Facilitation and Inhibition of Postural Responses
Through Controlled Sensory Input

The goal of treatment is to dampen (inhibit) abnormal postural reactions while fostering (facilitating) more normal and more efficient reactions, such as righting and equilibrium reactions. This is achieved by handling the infant and guiding his or her movements. Through handling, the therapist controls the sensory input to some degree and, in an indirect way, the motor output. This results in a more normal sensory feedback which enhances the establishment of normal automatic responses and the subsequent learning of effective voluntary movements without the need to drill these skills.

Inhibition of abnormal motor patterns and facilitation of more normal patterns as an automatic response to specific handling techniques was first described by Berta and Karel Bobath [6] as the fundamental concept of the neurodevelopmental treatment (NDT) approach. Mary Quinton [7] has adapted these principles specifically to very early treatment, e.g., intervention within the first 9 to 12 months of life.

GENERAL TREATMENT PRINCIPLES

Modification of Body Schema

Quality of motor behavior and learning of new motor skills depend on previous sensorimotor experiences and their internal representation which form the body schema. The body schema is shaped and continuously reshaped by sensorimotor experiences. Modification of abnormal motor behavior can, therefore, be achieved by modifying and improving the patient's body schema through selective sensory input which indirectly controls the motor output and determines type and quality of sensory feedback. This sensory feedback should reflect purposeful sensorimotor experiences.

It seems that sensory preparation in the form of mobile weight bearing on different body parts precedes their respective motor control. For example, the infant rests most of the body weight on head and upper trunk in prone and supine before developing control of head and shoulder girdle. Treatment should provide similar sensory preparations.

Grading of Stimulation

The therapist's goal of providing as much normal feedback as possible must never result in a bombardment of multiple and diverse stimuli. A systematic approach is recommended with room for ample repetition of appropriate postural responses in a variety of positions and situations. Nevertheless, the intervention program must still strive for a balance of multiple motor patterns. Exclusive reinforcement of one motor pattern over a longer period of time contrasts with the sequence of normal development and may have adverse effects.

The selective and graded support provided, permits the therapist to bring the infant into a variety of positions even when the infant has only minimal postural control. Depending on the support given, the demands placed on the infant's balancing skills can vary widely in any one position. For example, the infant with poor sitting balance can already be treated in supported standing as long as the therapist can provide proper postural alignment. Here, it should be pointed out that parents place their babies into various positions, such as supported standing, at a very early age and usually long before the infant has achieved the respective developmental milestone.

Components of Movement

The treatment plan reflects the sequence of normal development. Complex and skillful activities are based on a combination of simpler movement components acquired at an earlier stage of development. These motor components may be seen as "subskills," some of which encompass the activities described in this chapter (Specific Treatment Procedures). The therapist should provide a solid foundation of these early and basic subskills before working on more difficult motor tasks. Some of the most important basic skills are righting of head and trunk, and proximal stability of trunk, shoulder, and pelvic girdle. These require modification of primitive and total motor patterns.

Although functional activities are a major concern, this approach puts little stress on practicing these functional activities or developmental milestones per se. Instead it aims to provide the infant with the postural building blocks required for a variety of automatic and volitional activities. A well-founded knowledge of normal development allows the therapist to select subskills required for activities of current as well as future developmental skills and motor functions.

Dynamic Versus Static Treatment

Since the facilitation of righting and equilibrium reactions is a major goal of treatment, it follows that treatment must not be static but should always be dynamic. Every movement is prepared and combined with weight shift. Weight shift facilitates movement and can be used as a tool to elicit the desired postural reactions. A small amplitude of weight shift is often used to facilitate control of every phase of the activity.

The same approach is used when trying to increase mobility and achieve elongation of muscles. Passive stretch and forceful resistance are not used. Instead, motor responses are facilitated which themselves result in active elongation. The same process can be seen in normal development, for example, in the infant who rocks from side to side in the supine position with legs raised off the support which results in elongation of the extensors. Through small range movements and weight shifting the patient is prevented from building up abnormal tonus which would resist movement in the desired direction.

Individualized Programs

The therapist must be aware of the impact that therapeutic handling has on
the shaping of early sensorimotor experiences and the resulting body schema,
the very tools upon which later skills will be based. The motor patterns
which the therapist facilitates must, therefore, be as accurate and normal as
achievable for the individual infant. The need for thorough knowledge of
normal development and normal movement cannot be overemphasized. Relatively small deviations from the norm may prove to be limiting factors in
highly complex skills as they develop during later developmental stages. Instructions to parents must be precise and detailed to prevent abnormal compensations.

The implementation of the program and the application of handling techniques must also take into account individual differences. Reactions to stimuli and responses to various aspects of handling vary considerably, depending
for example on basic postural tonus. A play activity causing too much excitement and subsequent hypertonicity in one infant may not arouse another at
all. Tempo and rhythm of movements influence tonus. Very slow and rhythmical movements allow the hypotonic infant to stabilize with compensatory
patterns and to fall from one end position into the other. Very fast movements, on the other hand, do not provide sufficient time for postural adjustments in the hypertonic infant. Orientation toward gravity affects postural
tonus. With the hypotonic infant who sinks into gravity and who almost
melts to the support, postural tonus may improve drastically in more upright
positions. Given little support, these infants are forced to be more active
while the baby with predominantly high tonus tightens up even more when
feeling insecure. Amplitude of movements is another factor to take into
account. Postural control must be achieved in a small range before full balance can be expected during wide range movements.

Specific techniques of sensory stimulation such as approximation (cocontraction), tapping, vibration, etc., can change tonus drastically and need to be
applied with good judgment. From the result of the evaluation, the therapist
can predict to some degree the infant's reactions and can adjust handling
appropriately. The patient's response to being handled and moved determines what further input the therapist needs to provide. At all times the
therapist is guided by the patient's response.

Shaping Motor Behavior Through Handling

This approach uses "hands on" to elicit and shape motor responses. Touch in
itself is, of course, a stimulus and appropriate grading must be adjusted to the

individual. Very light touch is most stimulating and may cause withdrawal. A firm touch is preferable and is also more directive. It is, however, important not to provide undue pressure. It is not necessary nor desirable to embrace a patient with a tight grip. An open grip with extended fingers provides sufficient support and directive guidance. It also causes the pressure to be applied through the palm and/or long side of the fingers and prevents irritating localized pressure through the fingertips. In order to facilitate finely graded responses, the sensory input provided through the therapist's hands must be finely tuned and dynamic, that is, using variation of pressure through the various parts of the hand.

A bombardment of tactile input caused by frequent changes of hand placement can be very disorganizing and overwhelming for a sensitive infant. When the therapist distributes sensory cuing all over the baby's body by jumping from one contact point to another, the infant receives confusing messages and may consequently react with irritation and crying—and with reason. A constant and firm contact from very few points of control (key points) is desirable and seems most effective.

The therapist handles the infant not just for support but to provide guidance (facilitation) and correction (inhibition) of postural reactions. The point of control must therefore be carefully selected. Proximal points of control (i.e., trunk, shoulder, or pelvic girdle) permit the greatest impact on the motor patterns. Distal control is chosen as soon as the infant is capable of taking over a major part of postural control. The goal is of course to fade out the control provided by therapist or parent.

The amount of support and control is also adjusted to the individual infant. During balance activities the therapist should try to handle the infant mostly from the non-weight-bearing side to facilitate righting against gravity, while too much support on the weight-bearing side may encourage the infant to lean into gravity.

Holistic Approach

The motor dysfunction must be seen in perspective to the total child and the child-family situation. Treatment goals must stress funtions that are important to child and family. Intervention requires a multidisciplinary team in which the family plays a vital role.

SPECIFIC TREATMENT PROCEDURES

Treatment procedures are categorized according to motor functions and their major components rather than by diagnosis. The motor functions are described in order of increasing degrees of complexity.

In every activity the main focus is on postural alignment (integration of righting reactions), control and balance (function of equilibrium reactions), and the quality of individual movement components. Handling is described in detail to stress the importance of correct alignment and control. The techniques themselves are changeable and must be adapted to individual needs of patient, therapist, and parent. The selection of activities is limited and does not represent a complete treatment program. A concept for treatment and not a procedural outline is described here.

Some of the ideas underlying the following activities and handling techniques have been presented and generated during a neurodevelopmental treatment (NDT) course given by Mary Quinton and Elsbeth Kong in Seattle, Washington, and during an NDT baby course presented by Mary Quinton in Roosevelt, New York.

HEAD CONTROL

Early signs of abnormality may occur in patterns of head posture. Even the baby who manages to lift and balance the head may do so in an abnormal or immature fashion. Without controlled head orientation more complex motor functions and, indeed, learning about the self and the world is impeded.

Different degrees of head control and some typical abnormal compensations have been described in Chapter 4.

Righting into Flexion Against Gravity

Finely graded postural adjustments of head and trunk require a delicate balance between axial flexion and extension. When this balance is impaired, shoulder girdle and trunk cannot provide a stable base for the head to move upon. Midline control and lateral righting are consequently difficult. Elongation of the neck cannot take place. Instead, tightness in the neck and shoulder girdle area may lead to contractures.

Activity

Start at a point where good posture and balance of the head are easily achieved, such as supported sitting. Facing the therapist, the infant is tilted slowly back; the goal is to elicit proper alignment between head and trunk. When the center of gravity is shifted behind the base of support, the pelvis tilts posteriorly and the spine flexes evenly. At a certain point of recline, the baby may elevate and flex the legs as a balance reaction.

Handling

To correct the shoulder position, the therapist holds the infant around the shoulders while pulling gently downward and outward. Instead of moving the infant continually throughout the whole range of the movement, the therapist rocks the baby gently in small lateral and anterior/posterior excursions. When the head falls back into extension, the infant is brought into a more upright position. Pressure should be distributed on the shoulders over as broad an area as possible. The shoulders are very sensitive to sharp and pointed pressure, therefore, the therapist's or parent's fingers should be kept extended to prevent localized pressure from the fingertips (Figs. 1a and b).

Variations. Flexor control and neck elongation are further reinforced when toys are placed in front of the infant, or when the therapist or parent lies back with the infant straddled across the lap (Fig. 1c). In this position, weight shifting and lateral righting reactions (see below) can be induced through lateral weight shift of the therapist or parent.

Midline Orientation

Flexor control leads to midline orientation and bimanual activities, such as hand to hand, hand to mouth, knees or feet motion, or reaching for toys. Grasping and sucking may result in too much tonus (tightness around shoulder girdle), in which case the infant should be encouraged only to reach, swipe at, or hit objects until better control can be established.

Activity

Toys or other stimuli are presented in midline while the infant is in supported sitting as described in Righting into Flexion Against Gravity, or in a well aligned supine position.

Handling

Techniques of handling are described under activities in Righting into Flexion Against Gravity.

Lateral Head Righting

Lateral righting is an extremely important reaction which deserves high priority in the treatment of motor disabilities. It represents a major step beyond total flexion/extension and leads to rotation within the body axis which is an essential subskill for mature balance reactions. Some onset of lateral righting is obvious at an early stage of development (3 to 4 months).

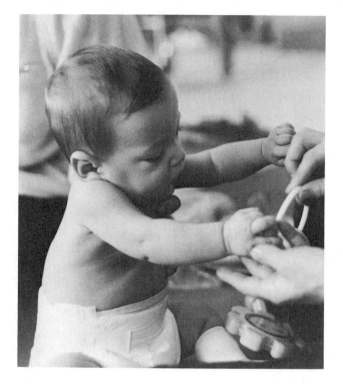

Figure 1a Head and shoulder girdle posture are severely impaired, causing the head to tilt slightly back and to one side while the shoulders are extremely elevated. (Photograph by Marion Madigan.)

In treatment, early facilitation of lateral righting prevents the infant from becoming locked into total and abnormal motor patterns.

Activity

The above activities are slightly modified. Instead of reclining the baby from sitting in a straight plane, lateral rocking and weight shifting are induced. The baby is rocked gently from side to side while tilted back. The amplitude of the lateral displacement must be adjusted to the infant's ability and may be very small at the beginning. With more lateral displacement, the trunk gradually rotates toward the non-weight-bearing side: the shoulder on the weight-bearing side is slightly forward in relation to the other shoulder. The infant who uses predominantly patterns of extension tends to rotate the trunk in

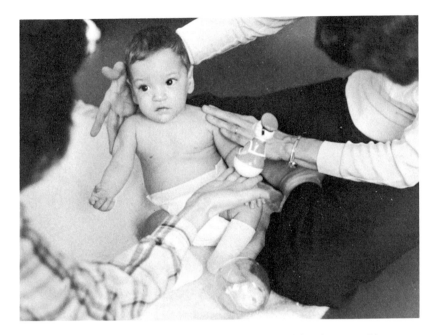

Figure 1b By stabilizing shoulder girdle and trunk with a downward/outward pull, the therapist can facilitate flexor control against gravity while tilting the infant back in sitting. The weight can be shifted to one side, by increasing pressure to the opposite shoulder in the direction of the weight shift; this facilitates lateral righting against gravity. Some downward pressure may also have to be maintained on the weight-bearing side to prevent improper shoulder elevation. (Photograph by Marion Madigan.)

the opposite direction. Proper frontal alignment between shoulder girdle and pelvis must be kept: the shoulder girdle should not be pulled sideways in relation to the pelvis.

Lateral righting combines lateral flexion and rotation toward the non-weight-bearing side with active elongation on the weight-bearing side.

Handling

From the non-weight-bearing side, the therapist elicits lateral flexion with downward traction through shoulder and arm while imposing a weight shift to the contralateral side (see Figs. 1b and c).

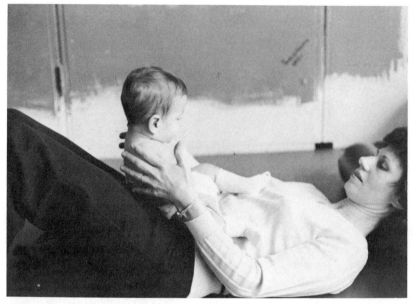

Figure 1c Neck elongation and head flexion can be encouraged by directing the infant's visual gaze accordingly. In this position, weight shifting and lateral righting can be induced through lateral movements of the therapist or parent. (Photograph by Marion Madigan.)

Neck Elongation and Shoulder Girdle Alignment

Lack of mobility in the neck and shoulder girdle area interferes with refined head control. While the neck muscles shorten, the shoulder girdle is elevated and tipped forward.

Activity

Supine. With fingers placed lengthwise over clavicle and acromion, the shoulder girdle is gradually rotated back, which leads to straightening of cervical and thoracic spine. The infant is encouraged to bring the arms forward to body or face, or toward the therapist's face, or to an object dangling from the therapist's neck.

Handling

The touch to the infant's shoulders must be gentle and not to the point of resistance. Sufficient time must be allowed for the infant to adapt. The direction of input is outward and slightly upward and backward. The arms are

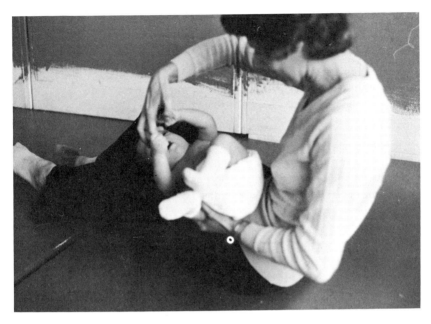

Figure 2 Body righting on head is facilitated by rolling the pelvis to one side. Proper postural alignment between head and shoulder girdle must be maintained. When turning the head too far, pronounced extension may occur and must be corrected. (Photograph by Marion Madigan.)

cradled between the forearms of the therapist. Once the shoulder girdle is aligned, pressure approximation can be directed throughout the trunk toward the pelvis to assist with proximal stability and caudal weight shift. The shoulder girdle is touched only on the top, the hands are not cupped around the shoulder joint to avoid compression.

Variation

The same method of handling can be applied in prone or prone on forearms. Care must be taken to not pull the shoulders too far back and to maintain the natural curvature of the thoracic spine.

Body Righting Reaction on Head

This ensures proper postural alignment and enables the baby to roll, for example, from supine toward the side or toward prone. Predominant exten-

sion and asymmetrical tonic neck reflex (ATNR) posturing as well as severe
hypotonicity may suppress the reaction.

Activities

The baby is placed in supine position with legs flexed. Body righting reaction
of the head is facilitated by rolling the pelvis toward either side. The baby
reacts by rolling the trunk and head toward the same side.

Handling

Scapular retraction and hyperextension of shoulders are inhibited through a
forward reach. With one or both hands on the pelvis, the therapist elicits
weight shift and turning to either side (Fig. 2). Elevation of the shoulder
girdle must be corrected (see Neck Elongation).

Carryover. To reinforce flexion against gravity, the parent is advised to
use the above position frequently for dressing. Some degree of rotation
between shoulder girdle and pelvis may evolve when, for example, removing
or putting on pants. This rotation prepares body righting reaction on body.

   To make active head flexion possible, the baby should be rolled halfway
to the side when pulled to a sitting position or being reclined to supine. Control is provided through arms or shoulder girdle as required.

TRUNK CONTROL

The development of head control overlaps the subsequent development of
trunk control. Free head movements are only possible with some stability
of shoulder girdle and trunk. Also, head movements elicit compensatory
movements of the trunk. In supine, the neck righting reaction causes the
baby to roll to the side when the head is turned. The neck righting reaction
is already present in the newborn and is well-developed by 4 months of age.
In prone, head and trunk move initially toward the side the baby turns to;
later on, as equilibrium develops, the body weight is shifted toward the opposite side which enables the infant to lift the non-weight-bearing hand and
reach toward objects within his or her field of vision. Intrinsic trunk movements as required for righting and balance reactions are first prepared in supine and in prone. Abnormal postural tonus and poorly integrated head control impede further development of trunk control.

Integration Between Flexion and Extension in Prone

Antigravity tonus through the trunk and a caudal weight shift are necessary
to support the head being lifted.

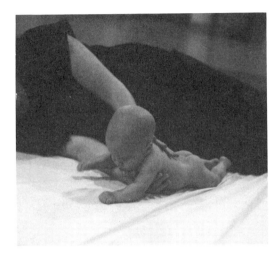

Figure 3a The therapist provides input for caudal weight shift and spinal extension by placing one hand across the infant's back while the hand across the chest maintains shoulder girdle and upper trunk alignment.

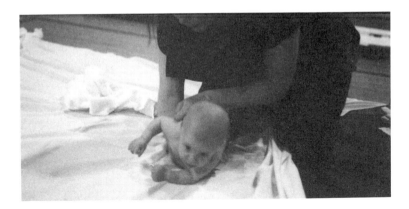

Figure 3b During weight shift to one side, the arm needs to stabilize while shoulder girdle and trunk rotate over.

Activity

The infant lies prone. The therapist assists caudal weight shift and spinal extension by handling from the trunk.

Handling

One hand is across the infant's chest, the other hand is across the back. Input on the chest must be gentle and aims at elongation rather than lifting. Weight shift and extension are elicited with caudal input to the spine (Fig. 3a).

Activity 2

Once sufficient trunk tonus is achieved, lateral weight shift can be elicited.

Handling

The weight shift input is not in a straight lateral plane. Instead, the direction of input is backward and to the opposite side to achieve axial rotation. Hand placement is as in activity 1 (Fig. 3b).

Variation

Handling from the shoulder girdle is described in the previous section (Neck Elongation and Shoulder Girdle Alignment).

Integration Between Flexion and Extension in Supine

Integration between flexion and extension enables the baby to keep the head in midline with good neck elongation, to extend the arms forward and to grasp knees or feet, and so forth. Initially, the knees are flexed due to the tendency toward total flexor patterns. Only when differentiation of movement patterns is possible, can the infant combine flexion of the hips with extension of the knees. With hands on knees or feet, the baby rocks from side to side which demonstrates highly developed abdominal control and is a direct preparation for sitting balance. This degree of abdominal action and control is often omitted in the handicapped infant and results in lack of mobility and lack of movement differentiation between hip, pelvis, and trunk.

Activity 1

In supine the infant lifts the legs with abduction and external rotation. When possible, reaching for legs or feet is included. During the activity, trunk and pelvis maintain a stable posture against the support surface. At all times the knees should be further apart than the feet.

Handling

The therapist cradles the lateral side of the infant's legs with hands flat and places fingers straight and behind, above, and below the knees. The feet are placed between the therapist's forearms. When dissociated movements between the pelvis and legs are difficult, the pelvis is stabilized with one hand while lifting only one leg. Pressure through the flexed leg into hip and pelvis established sufficient proximal stabilization to free the hand for lifting the other leg. Once the legs are flexed, a more distal point of control, such as the feet may be sufficient. If the infant needs help with reaching, the legs can be supported against the therapist's trunk. Input to shoulder girdle and arms has been described previously (Neck Elongation and Shoulder Girdle Alignment).

Activity 2

With the therapist's hands on the infant's knees or feet, the infant performs small amplitude rocking motions from side to side.

Handling

The therapist places her hands on the infant's flexed knees and lower legs. Pressure is placed toward the hips. If need be, the therapist uses her extended fingers to support the infant's hands. Weight shift is achieved by leaning strongly to one side. Care must be taken, not to pull the contralateral leg into adduction. In order to avoid eliciting undue extension, the contralateral side must not be lifted by the therapist. Instead, rotation should occur in response to the weight shift.

Righting Reactions of Head and Trunk in Sitting

Integration between flexion and extension in prone and in supine prepare trunk control in sitting. Before full integration between flexion and extension is developed, the baby sits in a ring sitting fashion: the legs are abducted and flexed at hips and knees, similar to the pattern assumed in supine during early hand to foot activities. By 9 to 10 months of age, the infant has sufficiently practiced differentiated leg movements in supine to be able to sit in a variety of postures with good sitting balance.

The hypotonic baby often sits with the legs in pronounced flexion/abduction and with an anterior pelvic tilt. With the trunk in front of the line of gravity, abdominal muscles are not activated for balancing and lateral righting is inhibited. In this case, head and trunk control must be prepared in supported sitting, prone, and supine as described above.

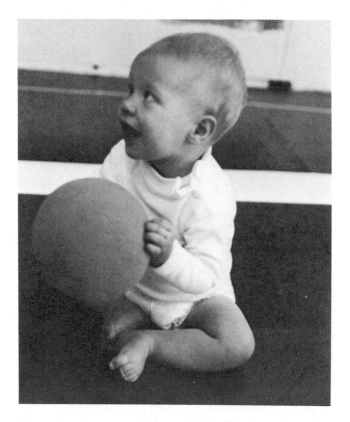

Figure 4a The extremely flexed and abducted posture of the legs interferes with the development of proper sitting balance. Stress is seen in the tight curling of the toes. (Photograph by Carol Herwig.)

Alternatively, the pelvis is tilted too far back due to lack of control or mobility. The activities described in the previous section (Integration of Flexion and Extenion in Supine) are an excellent preparation for better sitting posture and balance.

The infant who has developed some degree of head and trunk control can be further challenged in righting and balancing while sitting.

Activities

In sitting, the baby is handled from the pelvis while the therapist displaces the center of gravity in every direction (Figs. 4a and b).

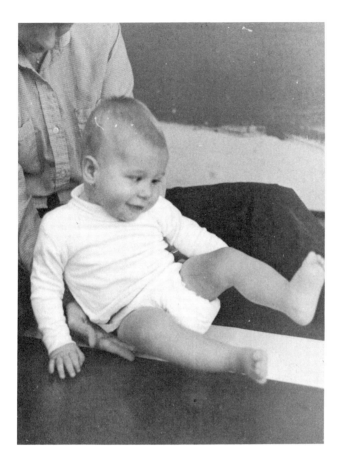

Figure 4b By handling the infant from the pelvis, the therapist can displace the center of gravity in every direction. To achieve axial rotation, the therapist should rotate the left side of this infant's pelvis backward. (Photograph by Carol Herwig.)

Handling

The therapist, sitting either behind or in front of the infant, places both hands on the dorsal side of pelvis and hips while tilting the baby slightly back so that the shoulders are behind the hips. The weight is shifted laterally while rotating the contralateral side back. When an additional stimulus for lateral trunk righting is necessary, the therapist applies a caudally directed pull from the lower ribcage using the base or lateral side of the thumb. Initially,

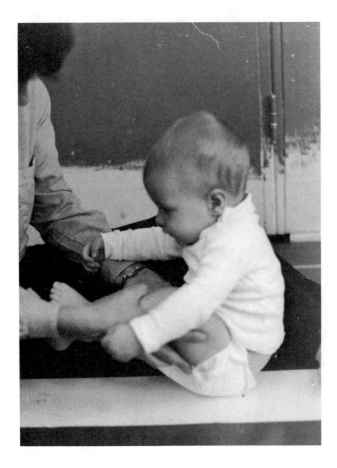

Figure 4c   After some sitting balance is established, the infant can be handled from the legs (with a pillow behind the back, just in case!). (Photograph by Carol Herwig.)

lateral oscillations should be minimal. When the infant is challenged beyond his or her limits, abnormal postural fixation may occur around the shoulders, arms, and neck. With increased lateral weight shift, the infant may place the hands down for propping.

When less assistance is required, the infant can be handled from knees or feet (Fig. 4c).

Variations. When proper trunk righting cannot be elicited using handling from pelvis and legs, the therapist places her hands along each side of the trunk and guides the infant through the proper weightshift and rotation.

ROLLING AND BELLY CRAWLING

Mature patterns of rolling as well as normal patterns of belly crawling require a number of similar movement components. These include weight shifting through shoulder girdle, trunk, and pelvis, with active elongation on the weight-bearing side; lateral righting of head and trunk toward the non-weight-bearing side, and rotation within the body axis. All these movement components are reflected in the amphibian reaction where the weight-bearing side of the trunk elongates relatively to the non-weight-bearing side. At the same time, both limbs on the weight-bearing side extend and adduct while both on the other side flex. Excessive flexion or extension throughout the body inhibits the amphibian reaction, although many of these infants learn to roll or crawl but do so in an abnormal fashion.

Better function and quality of posture and movements can be prepared by facilitating the amphibian reaction as well as encouraging rotation within the body axis.

Amphibian Reaction

Appropriate elongation on the weight-bearing side is hampered by tightness in the shoulder girdle, especially between scapula and humerus. Full overhead flexion of the weight-bearing shoulder is inhibited by scapular protraction and internal rotation of the shoulder.

Activities

The infant lies prone with both shoulders fully flexed and in slight external rotation. The arms rest on the supporting surface in neutral abduction or slight adduction. While the weight is shifted to one side, elongation of the weight-bearing side is initiated from chest and shoulder. Full flexion of the shoulder is rendered through a combination of shoulder, scapular, and spinal

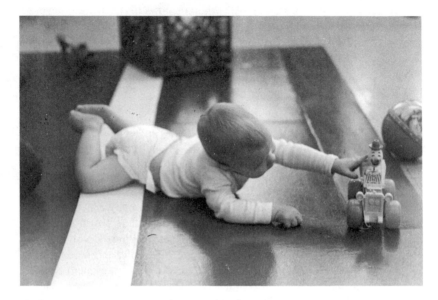

Figure 5a In contrast with the normal postural adjustments (amphibian re-action), head and trunk are flexed on the weight-bearing side—into gravity—while this infant reaches forward. Abduction of the limbs interferes with lateral weight shift.

movement. Lack of mobility in the shoulder is often compensated for by excessive spinal extension. This must be corrected by aligning shoulder and pelvis. Proper weight shifting and lateral righting are further accentuated with reinforcement of the external rotation of the weight-bearing shoulder (Figs. 5a and b).

Resistance to full shoulder flexion is never counteracted by pulling on the arm. Sensory acceptance and preparation of tonus for this position are achieved when the infant is slightly rolled over the weight-bearing arm with the shoulder flexed to a degree which is comfortable. The therapist rotates the infant's shoulder back and accentuates weight bearing on arm and scap-ula with downward pressure in the side-lying position.

Note: The hypotonic and hypermobile infant may lack proper response of the leg on the weight-bearing side. Instead of turning the leg so that the foot points forward when reaching side-lying position, the infant may maintain an

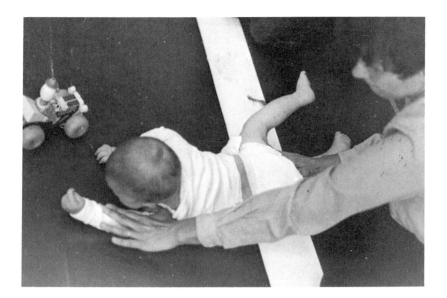

Figure 5b Lateral weight shift and amphibian reaction can be facilitated by moving the weight-bearing arm into external rotation and adduction and maintaining the weight-bearing leg in external rotation and extension. The shoulder must be completely flexed (no space between axilla and support). (Photograph by Carol Herwig.)

extreme degree of external rotation. More often, internal rotation occurs preventing extension of the hip. This must be corrected and proper postural adjustments need to be facilitated. Normally, the weight-bearing leg is maintained in extension and external rotation, yet it turns in accordance with the turning of the pelvis. Better support tonus on the weight-bearing leg is stimulated when the sensory feedback is accentuated by the therapist pushing the infant's leg and foot against the support.

Handling

To correct scapular protraction, the infant is handled from the shoulder girdle. The sensory feedback of weight bearing on the lateral surface of scapula and humerus is accentuated with firm downward pressure. Lateral righting can be facilitated by a slight pull in a caudal direction which is applied to the scapula and upper trunk of the non-weight-bearing side.

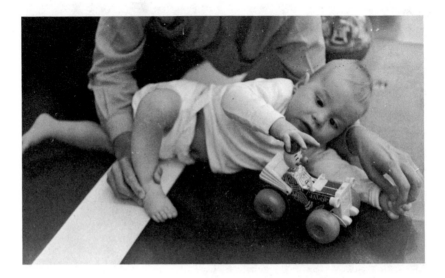

Figure 5c While the infant plays in the side-lying position, the parent is shown how to facilitate proper upper extremity weight bearing while encouraging weight bearing on the contralateral foot. Note weight bearing on the lateral part of the foot due to external rotation of the hip (compare with Fig. 12b, Chap. 4). (Photograph by Carol Herwig.)

Variations. The amphibian reaction can also be facilitated from both limbs on the weight-bearing side or from the weight-bearing arm and contralateral leg (Fig. 5c).

When the above handling method does not produce sufficient trunk and hip flexion, the therapist changes hand placement to the weight-bearing shoulder and the opposite side of the trunk (Fig. 5d).

Carryover The mother is instructed occasionally to place or carry the infant in side-lying position (see Chap. 7) to reinforce the amphibian reaction.

Rotation Within Body Axis

Patterns of proper weight shift and lateral righting have been discussed for the supine, prone, and sitting positions (see activities for Lateral Head Right-

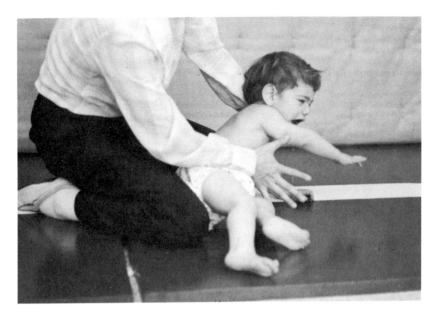

Figure 5d Rolling from prone to side lying, supine, or sitting is facilitated from the low rib cage and abdomen. To prevent shoulder and arm retraction on the non-weight-bearing side, the therapist extends fingers against the back of the infant's arm. This point of control is also used to shift the weight forward and to elicit rolling toward prone. At the same time the therapist retards the forward movement of the pelvis with the palm of the hand and thus encourages rotation within body axis. (Photograph by Carol Herwig.)

ing, Integration Between Flexion and Extension in Prone, Righting of Head and Trunk in Sitting, and Amphibian Reaction). Lateral righting and rotation within the body axis are also encouraged by placing the infant in a side-lying position. Patterns of extension and flexion are balanced allowing lateral flexion of the spine. When the infant moves toward prone, extension increases; when moving toward supine, flexion against gravity increases. "Body righting on body" leads to rotation and segmental rolling. When the fine interplay between flexion and extension is disturbed, postural alignment and balance during rolling are disturbed.

Activities

The side-lying position is a good way to start facilitation of segmental rolling. Initially, the excursions toward supine and prone are small. To prevent excessive extension of the spine, the shoulders lead when rolling toward prone, and the pelvis leads when rolling toward supine. The non-weight-bearing leg moves into flexion, external rotation and adduction of the hip while rolling toward supine, and into extension, external rotation and abduction while rolling toward prone. The weight-bearing arm is in alignment with the trunk: in full shoulder flexion and in some degree of external rotation.

Handling

Rotation of pelvis against shoulder girdle in prone to supine or side lying to sitting is facilitated from the lower rib cage and abdomen.

UPPER EXTREMITY WEIGHT BEARING

Upper extremity functions, such as reaching, controlled arm movements in space and, finally, manipulative skills require dynamic postural stability of the shoulder girdle on a stable trunk and dissociation of movement between head, shoulder girdle, and arms. These skills develop initially during activities of weight bearing. Some patterns of normal and abnormal upper extremity weight bearing are described in Chapter 4 (Patterns of Upper Extremity Weight Bearing). Efficient patterns of upper extremity weight bearing in prone are based on the ability to shift weight through trunk and pelvis. Without active hip extension, it is difficult to stabilize the pelvis for proper weight shifting.

Pelvic Control and Hip Extension in Prone

When head and chest are raised off the support, active hip extension is apparent, first fleetingly and then more consistently by 5 to 6 months. Hip extension in space, such as lifting of the legs in prone, or in ventral suspension is a developmentally higher skill and develops later (6 to 8 months). The infant with delayed motor development keeps the hips in flexion and bears weight mostly on the chest while prone, and reaching activities are therefore hampered. In this case, weight bearing and weight shifting through the pelvis should be encouraged.

Activity

The infant is placed prone with shoulders externally rotated and fully flexed. The therapist is positioned in front of the infant, holding arms or hands, while encouraging the infant to lift head and chest off the support. The goal is to achieve a visible contraction of the glutei muscles. The infant should not be kept in a static posture. Small lateral weight shifts or rotation of head and trunk can be easily facilitated, especially when the infant lies on a large ball. Also, one arm may be brought down for propping while the infant is encouraged to reach with the other hand. Observe proper head righting with elongation of the neck.

Handling

The more distally the infant is held, and the less support is given, the more weight bearing occurs through the hips. When possible, the therapist supports the infant from the hands. The palms of the hands are turned slightly toward each other to achieve external rotation at the shoulders. The infant should not use the distal support as a point of fixation, which may lead to a pull into flexion from the arms. When more support is needed, the infant is held more proximally, that is, by the shoulders and trunk. Elevation and protraction of shoulder and scapula can be inhibited and external rotation of the shoulder facilitated by encompassing shoulder girdle and arm.

Dissociation of Movements Between Shoulder Girdle, Head, and Trunk

The infant with sensorimotor deficit often lacks the ability to dissociate movements between head, shoulder girdle, and trunk. Weight shift is often initiated from the head. The shoulder girdle cannot be stabilized and the scapula is thus pulled into protraction and elevation during arm and/or head movements. Appropriate righting of head and trunk is now inhibited.

Activity

The infant lies prone on forearms or hands on a mat, roll, or over the therapist's lap. Lateral weight shift through the trunk is facilitated by pushing in a diagonal direction, from one shoulder toward the opposite hip (Figs. 6a and b).

Handling

With both hands on the infant's chest and with extended fingers leaning against the frontal and upper part of the shoulder girdle, the therapist can correct scapular protraction and modify trunk responses.

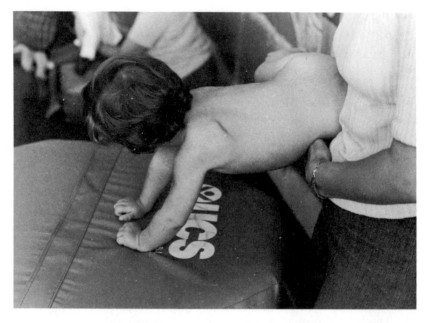

Figure 6a   Poor shoulder girdle stability is indicated in the winging of the scapula. The posture of the left arm suggests some ATNR influence: the elbow is slightly flexed in combination with scapular protraction. The trunk sinks into gravity. (Photograph by Carol Herwig.)

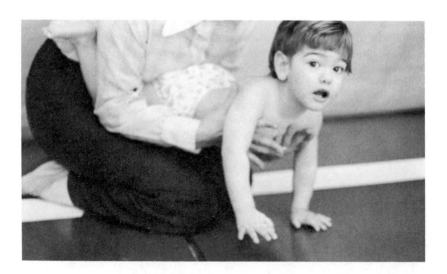

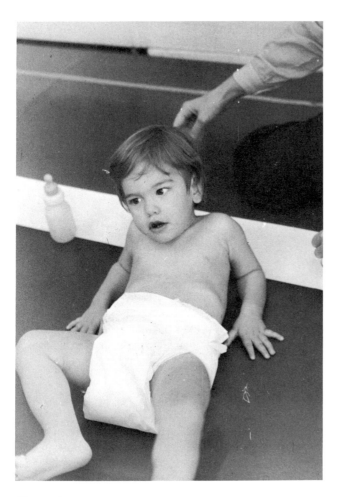

Figure 7a Poor shoulder girdle stability is especially obvious in supine on arms and is combined with an inactive, "sagging" posture of the trunk. Note the flaring of the ribs due to inactivity of the abdominal muscles. Compare with Figure 7b. (Photograph by Carol Herwig.)

Figure 6b In prone on hands, better integration between flexion and extension can be facilitated by supporting the infant under the chest. With this point of control the therapist can also facilitate lateral trunk righting reactions when weight is shifted to one side. Support can be given at the lateral margin of the scapula. (Photograph by Carol Herwig.)

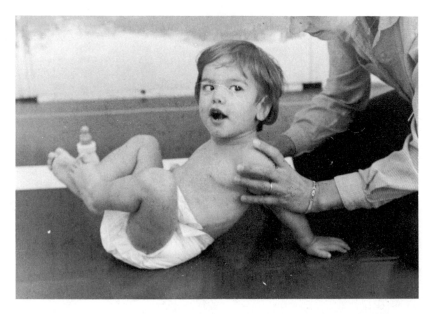

Figure 7b In order to achieve active control of shoulder girdle and trunk, the infant is handled from the shoulders. Compare with Figure 7a. (Photograph by Carol Herwig.)

Upper Extremity Weight Bearing in Reclined Sitting

Activity

Proper patterns of weight bearing on elbows or hands and weight shifting can also be carried out with the infant in reclined sitting. In this position, the infant is encouraged to flex the head while extending the upper trunk. The therapist should inhibit any tendency to scapular protraction and pronounced internal rotation of the shoulders. Upper extremity weight bearing should be carried out in various degrees of shoulder rotation. This helps to also prepare protective extension of the arms backward where the shoulder is usually in a slight degree of internal rotation.

Handling

From shoulder girdle and upper trunk, the therapist can inhibit scapular protraction, accentuate weight bearing, and facilitate spinal extension and lateral weight shift. After correcting the should girdle alignment, the input is directed toward the pelvis to activate the trunk (Figs. 7a, b, and c).

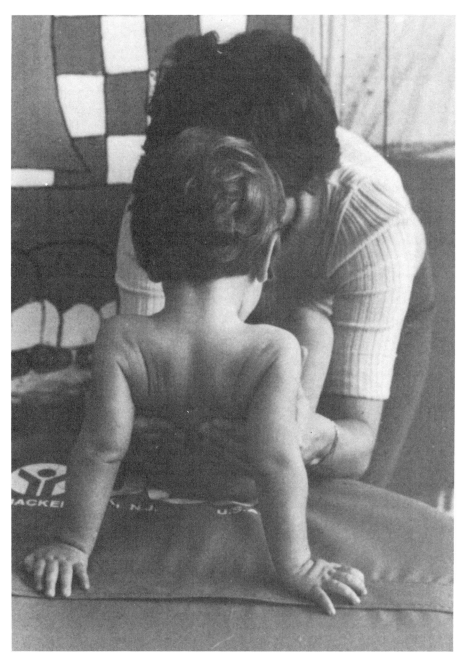

Figure 7c Active trunk extension is facilitated while the infant is encouraged to right in the direction of flexion against gravity. (Photograph by Carol Herwig.)

PROTECTIVE EXTENSION OF THE ARMS

Motor components required for protective extension are controlled extension against gravity and good stability of the shoulder girdle combined with mobility, and sufficient support tonus of the arms. Activities recommended in the section of upper extremity weight bearing prepare for protective extension of the arms. While the handicapped infant may prop on the hands, proper postural adjustments of head and trunk are lacking, especially in combination with lateral weight shifting. Shoulder girdle posture is also frequently impaired. The response may be delayed and support tonus of the arms is often insufficient.

Dynamic Stability of the Shoulder Girdle

Moving the trunk around the weight-baring arm is good preparation for the interplay between stability and mobility of shoulder girdle and arm.

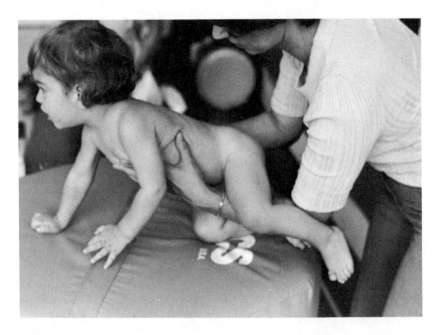

Figure 8a With the support under the chest and abdomen, flexion, lateral flexion, or rotation of the trunk can be facilitated. (Photography by Carol Herwig.)

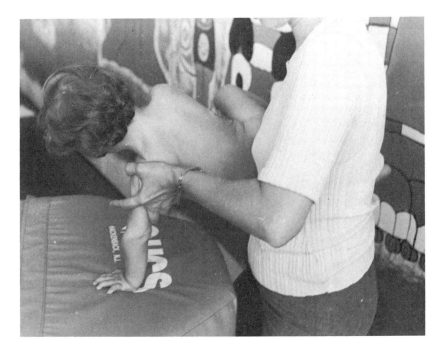

Figure 8b Grasping the infant around the shoulder allows the therapist to correct posture of the shoulder girdle and arm. (Photograph by Carol Herwig.)

Activity

With support under the chest and the abdomen, the infant is held in ventral suspension while leaning on both hands. The therapist induces lateral weight shift with axial rotation. During every phase of the activity, proper head righting must be facilitated and any tendency toward scapular protraction must be corrected. Shoulder girdle control is especially difficult when all the weight is resting on one hand as when turning from prone on hands to supine on hands (Figs.6a, 8a to d).

Handling

The therapist gives support with one hand under chest and abdomen in order to monitor trunk responses, e.g., flexion, lateral flexion, elongation. The other hand is placed on the weight-bearing shoulder with the thumb on the ventral side of the shoulder to correct scapular protraction and elevation.

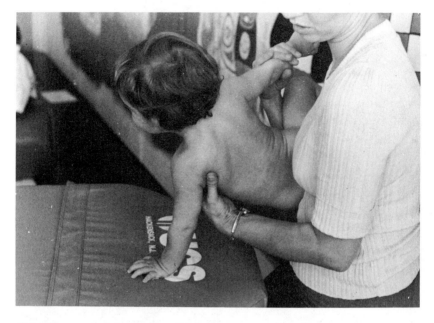

Figure 8c During the activity the therapist gradually reduces support and leaves more control to the infant. (Photography by Carol Herwig.)

The extended fingers lean against the infant's elbow to prevent collapsing of the arm, while the antithenar leans against the lateral margin of the scapula to inhibit pronounced abduction and winging of the scapula.

Variations. In prone as well as in side propping, the infant can be encouraged to reach in different directions, including crossing of the midline.

 When some shoulder girdle stability has been achieved, support from the upper trunk may be sufficient and can be substituted for direct handling of the infant from the shoulder girdle and arm.

 Protective extension should be elicited in all positions and the therapist should vary speed and direction of displacement. Depending on the degree of postural control, the infant is handled from either proximal or distal points.

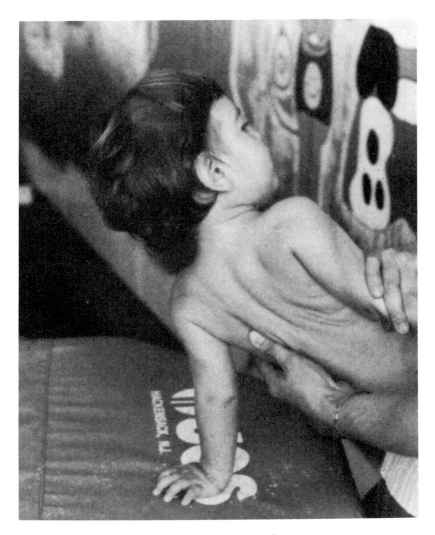

Figure 8d Therapy must be dynamic and should consist of movement sequences, such as prone on hands to side propping to supine on hands and back. The difficulty of the task changes consistently and the therapist should be guided by the infant's response. For example, the further the body is shifted over the weight-bearing arm (forward, sideways), the greater the challenge. (Photography by Carol Herwig.)

FOURPOINT CRAWLING

Fourpoint crawling is another big step in the infant's attempt to raise off the floor. It requires differentiation of movements and—with the pelvis off the floor—advanced skills of balancing. By the time the baby assumes fourpoint kneeling (by about 7 to 8 months), equilibrium reactions have emerged in prone, supine, and possibly in sitting. Before fourpoint crawling becomes an efficient means of locomotion, the infant has practiced balance by rocking in all directions while on hands and knees.

The infant with poor postural control keeps the center of gravity low while bearing most of his or her weight on the legs. This inhibits lateral weight shift and reciprocal leg movements.

To encourage proper crawling patterns, balance reactions are facilitated in fourpoint-kneeling (Figs. 9a-c).

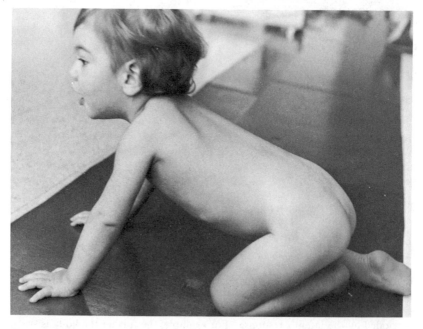

Figure 9a With pronounced hip flexion, weight bearing occurs predominantly on the legs, which inhibits lateral weight shift and frequently results in a pattern of "bunny hopping."

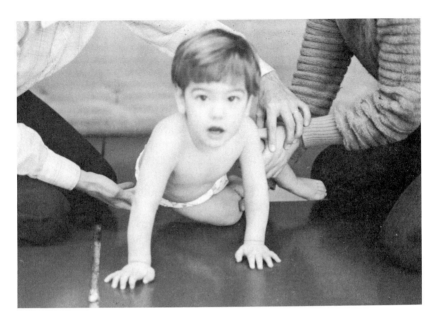

Figure 9b By correcting the leg posture, the parent can facilitate lateral weight shifting and axial rotation to prepare for reciprocal crawling. (Photograph by Carol Herwig.)

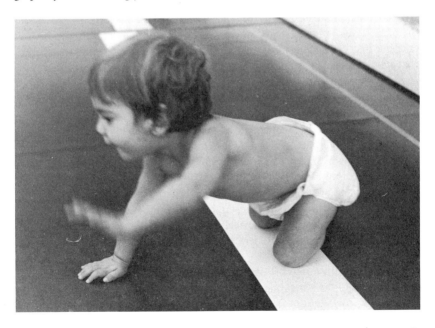

Figure 9c More appropriate postural tonus is indicated in improved postural alignment, balance, and distribution of weight bearing (compare with Fig. 9a). (Photograph by Carol Herwig.)

Pelvic Control and Balance Reactions in Fourpoint-Kneeling

Activity

The infant is placed on knees and hands with the legs in neutral abduction; knees under the body, and with knees and hips at about 90 degrees flexion. The therapist stabilizes the leg to which the weight is shifted and displaces the infant's center of gravity from the ventral side of trunk and pelvis or from the contralateral leg (Fig. 9b). Initially, the weight shift may be very small; later on, the infant can be moved between side sitting and quadruped position. Attention must be focused on adequate stability of the shoulder girdle and on proper rotation of pelvis and trunk. Any tendency to shoulder protraction must be discouraged. The weight-bearing arm should be vertical and especially during rotation, the shoulder should not move sideways in relation to the weight-bearing hand (see activities for Dissociation of Movements Between Shoulder Girdle, Head, and Trunk, and Dynamic Stability of the Shoulder Girdle for handling techniques).

STANDING AND WALKING

Ambulation is a major concern to parents of infants with developmental delay. To help parents deal with this anxiety, the therapist should discuss with them the developmental stages infants must pass through before they can take the first unassisted steps. It is often difficult for a lay person to accept that standing balance is not encouraged by placing the infant incessantly in an abnormal standing posture or being bounced on stiff legs. This may cause even further delay of balanced standing, especially when abnormal postural tonus is reinforced.

The fastest route to independent walking follows the course of normal development. Developmental stages of normal and abnormal patterns of standing and walking have been discussed in Chapter 4 (Patterns of Standing, Supported, Unsupported). In addition to the development of balance of head, trunk, and pelvis, the normal infant prepares the feet for weight bearing in various positions other than standing. When the infant finally pulls to standing, feet have acquired the necessary postural stability to carry the body weight while maintaining sufficient mobility to allow the gradual emergence of balance reactions.

The infant with poor postural tonus and abnormal motor patterns is frequently pulled into a standing position before the feet are properly prepared for the task. As a result, the weight distribution through the foot is abnormal, which in turn, affects the postural alignment of the body. Activities which encourage sensory awareness as well as balance reactions of the feet carried out in various positions other than standing help to diminish postural maladjustments in standing and walking. In addition, weight bearing in different degrees of hip and knee flexion (e.g., in the "bear position": standing on feet and hands), is especially helpful for the infant who tends to push into extreme extension or who locks the knees in hyperextension to achieve postural stability.

Foot-Eye Coordination

Normal infants (5 to 6 months old) engage in play activities with their feet while supine (legs in the air). They touch and handle feet, put toes into their mouths for investigation, and observe foot movements. The infant who lacks sufficient flexion against gravity is robbed of these opportunities. The developmentally delayed infant should be assisted in similar experiences and therapists should advise parents on how to incorporate "foot play" activities into their handling of the baby.

Activities

  1. To facilitate lifting of the legs, the infant lies well-supported on the parent's lap or on a mat. To maintain the feet in the infant's visual field requires a combination of flexor and extensor patterns. Excessive hip flexion combined with abduction must be modified. The infant is encouraged to reach and touch feet and/or place toes in mouth. It is important to observe and inhibit any increased flexor tonus that would pull the pelvis off the support. When excessive flexor tonus occurs in hands and arms, the baby is encouraged to touch the feet with open hands instead of grasping them.

  2. Sensory awareness of the feet can also be reinforced when the infant is assisted in grasping soft objects, such as a small rubber or foam ball, using the feet. To enhance tactile and proprioceptive feedback, the therapist helps the infant to move the object between the feet. For correction of abnormal foot alignment see Handling in the following section.

Weight Bearing on the Feet in Different Positions

Activities

Prone. Numerous prone positions lend themselves to weight bearing on dorsiflexed toes, for example, prone propping, pivoting in prone, belly crawling, amphibian reaction (weight-bearing leg). In all these positions, the leg is extended, the ankle and the toes are dorsiflexed. The same posture is used, later on, for the push off phase in walking and represents a high level of postural differentiation. This posture contrasts sharply with the abnormal patterns of weight bearing on the toes where the ankle is in plantar flexion.

Handling

The therapist brings the infant's toes into dorsiflexion, while elongating the heel to achieve good dorsiflexion of the ankle. Pronounced forefoot pronation must be corrected. From the heel, gentle pressure is applied to reinforce weight bearing on the toes. It is absolutely essential that the foot be well-aligned when techniques of cocontraction are applied.

Side-lying position. The normally developing infant often plays in side position on elbow or hand while using the upper, flexed leg for propping to give better postural stability (see Fig. 12b in Chapter 4). In this posture, the hip is in external rotation which allows weight bearing on the lateral border of the foot. This results in active lengthening of the lateral part of the foot while it encourages active lifting of the longitudinal arch of the foot.

The infant with sensorimotor deficits, if able to assume this position, uses internal rotation of the hip which leads to weight bearing on the medial border of the foot.

Handling

To encourage lengthening of the lateral and active shortening of the medial part of the foot, the therapist places the thumb against the medial surface of the calcaneus and the extended fingers against the lateral surface of the forefoot and the little toe. Any tendency toward internal rotation of the hip must be inhibited (see Fig. 5c).

Sitting. Partial weight bearing on the feet occurs in different sitting positions, especially in combination with weight shifting. When sitting on (note, not between!) the heels, the feet support almost the whole body weight (see Fig. 31 in Chap. 4). In this position the feet may be in plantarflexion or dorsiflexion of ankle and toes (see activity for Prone). Weight bearing on the feet can also be encouraged while the infant sits on a small stool or roll.

Handling

The therapist holds the infant's feet as described for activity for side-lying position. With the baby's feet well-aligned, the therapist bounces them repeatedly on the floor reinforcing proper weight bearing on the heel, lateral part of the forefoot, and all toes.

Balance Reactions of the Feet

Activity

In normal development, balance reactions of the feet are displayed in many different positions. Balance reactions of the feet deserve some attention in therapy, and should be encouraged during rolling, weight shifting in sitting, fourpoint kneeling, knee sitting, and so forth.

Handling

Different techniques of tapping can be applied either to the dorsiflexors of the ankle or to the plantar side of the toes to encourage dorsiflexion of the forefoot in combination with the appropriate balance reaction of the leg (abduction and flexion of the hip). Be careful not to elicit a positive support reaction by tapping on the ball of the foot.

Weight Bearing in Flexed Positions

Balance in standing and walking requires the ability to activate antigravity muscles while they are put into a state of dynamic elongation. This is difficult for a child with disturbed postural adjustments. Balance activities carried out in the "bear position," as on hands and feet, facilitate this skill and are, therefore, a good preparation for standing balance. The degree of flexion of the hips and knees should be varied during the activity.

Activity

The therapist sits on the mat, with the infant, facing away, and on lap. Holding the infant around the knees, the therapist shifts the infant's weight forward and thus facilitates leaning on the hands. In this position, the baby is rocked in all directions, in straight planes as well as in diagonal directions, to encourage lateral righting and rotation within body axis (Figs. 10a and b).

Handling

The therapist puts one arm on each side of the infant's trunk and places the hands around the infant's knees to allow (a) the body weight to be shifted forward, which increases dorsiflexion of the ankles (one or two fingers are placed behind the knee); (b) inhibition of plantarflexion by providing downward pressure from the thigh (with the palm of the hand); (c) extension of the knees by pivoting the pelvis upwards and forwards (with the fingers placed underneath the thighs). Note that the knees should not be pushed into total extension, this leads to possible locking of the knees in hyperex-

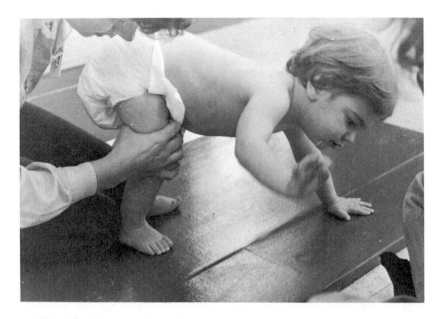

Figure 10a Balance activities in the plantigrade position elicit activation of muscles while they are in a state of dynamic elongation. (Photograph by Carol Herwig.)

tension and to passive standing, and (d) inhibition of adduction of the legs (with thumbs on medial surface of thigh and knee).

Variation. When foot alignment needs correcting, the therapist supports the feet with extended fingers while leaning the wrist or underarm on the infant's knees for control of the legs.

Standing Balance

Normally, an infant spends much time in supported standing, shifting the weight from foot to foot, twisting the body while letting go with one hand, or swinging one leg while trying to balance. Also, the infant can bend over to pick up a toy or sit down. All these activities are preparations for independent walking. For the handicapped infant, standing experiences are often static. Body and legs stiffen and do not allow adequate balance responses. It is, therefore, important that the therapist provide such an infant with the experience of dynamic standing together with appropriate postural support and control.

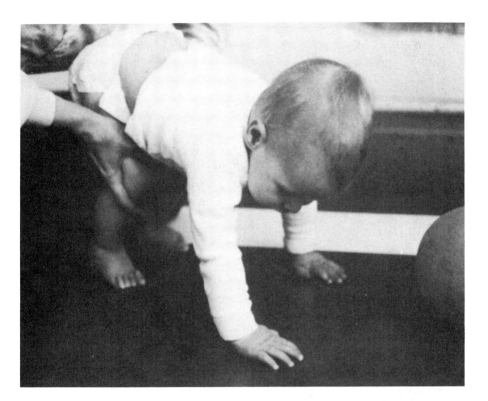

Figure 10b Weight shifting is facilitated in all directions. For a description of different handling techniques, see Handling for Standing Balance. (Photograph by Carol Herwig.)

Activity

Sitting on the mat, with the infant standing straddled over one leg, allows the therapist to modify support given to the infant by lowering or raising leg, grading the degree of hip and knee flexion when the infant sits down, or lifting the infant into the air when the standing posture deteriorates. Undue hip adduction is also inhibited. In the standing position, the infant is gently pushed in all directions either through movement of the therapist's leg or through handling. During weight shifting it is important to facilitate proper rotation, for example, trunk and pelvis rotate forward on the weight-bearing side (Figs. 11a to d). In standing, the degree of hip rotation and abduction influences the foot posture. Hip adduction combined with internal rotation

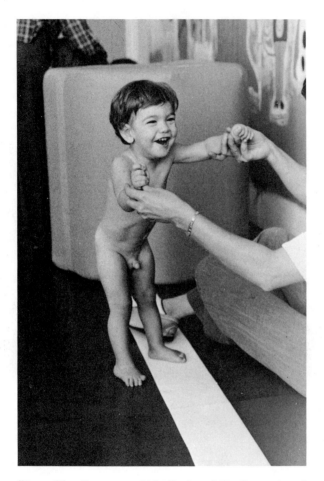

Figure 11a Pronounced hip flexion shifts the center of gravity far back in relation to the base of support (feet). (Photograph by Carol Herwig.)

leads to weight bearing on the medial part of the foot. Pronounced external rotation also shifts the weight to the medial part of the foot. Internal rotation and flexion of the hip tend to shift the weight predominantly to the toes.

   In treatment, the therapist facilitates a pattern of neutral or slight external rotation of the hips, unless the infant is in a step position where one leg assumes some degree of external rotation/abduction just before the push off phase.

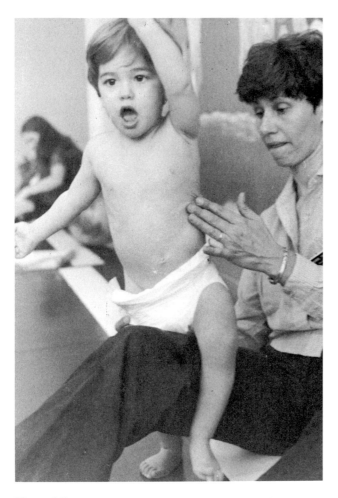

Figure 11b Hip extension is facilitated directly from the hip joint while the infant is also encouraged to rotate the non-weight-bearing side of trunk and pelvis backward. When corrective support to the trunk is given on the weight-bearing side, the infant may lean into gravity rather than actively to right against gravity as happens when handled from the non-weight-bearing side. (Photograph by Carol Herwig.)

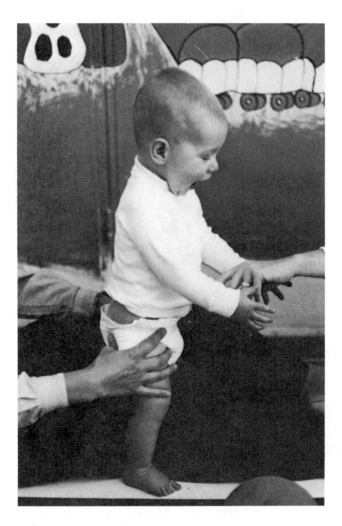

Figure 11c By straddling the infant over one leg during balance activities in standing, the therapist or parent can correct undue hip adduction, elicit lateral weight shift, or provide some standing support. Note well-integrated postural alignment throughout. (Photograph by Carol Herwig.)

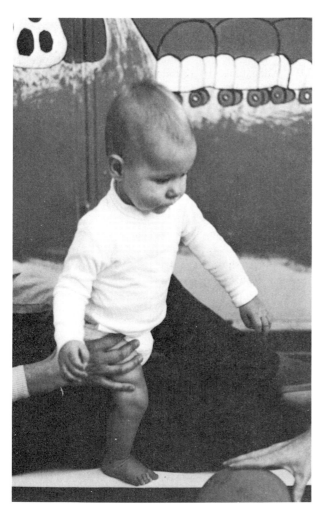

Figure 11d The step position over the therapist's leg facilitates axial rotation and external rotation of the hip. (Photograph by Carol Herwig.)

Handling

The point of control asserted by the therapist depends on the infant's level of postural control. The more distal the point of handling, the greater the degree of balance required. When poor foot alignment cannot be corrected bilaterally, the infant is brought to supported standing on one leg with the other knee leaning and bearing weight on the therapist's leg.

Variation. Turning the infant 90 degrees, places the baby in step position over the therapist's leg, which permits weight shifting forward and backward (see Fig. 11d).

Facilitation of Walking

Correction of an abnormal gait pattern and facilitation of normal walking require analysis and knowledge of the normal gait pattern. Walking requires a constant change in weight bearing. Before the initial step is taken, the weight must be shifted to one leg to free the other leg for the swing phase. In the mature gait pattern, the weight shift to one leg occurs with axial rotation: the weight-bearing side rotates forward, while the non-weight-bearing side rotates backward. Next, the weight is transferred forward. This occurs on the weight-bearing side, which means that the leg swings forward while the pelvis rotates backward on this side until the heel strikes the ground. Now, a diagonal weight shift occurs, leading, again, to a forward rotation on the weight-bearing side combined with the backward rotation on the other side. The rotation of the shoulder girdle describes a larger amplitude and results, therefore, in some counterrotation between pelvis and shoulder girdle.

This degree of rotation within the body axis is absent during the infant's initial stages of unassisted walking. However, rotation within the body axis is practiced by the infant in supported standing even before venturing to take a first unassisted step. During facilitation of walking it seems acceptable to introduce a slight degree of rotation, since the infant is given support. Careful grading of rotation is necessary to achieve proper postural alignment.

Handling

There are many ways of facilitating walking. The techniques used depend on the patient's skill in balance and postural alignment. It is not feasible here to describe more than one facilitation technique.

Substantial postural control can be achieved when the therapist walks behind the infant holding the shoulders and/or chest. For additional support and control, the therapist can use the legs pressed against the infant's hips

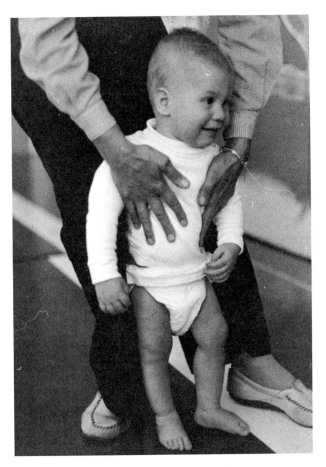

Figure 12 When substantial guidance and support are needed during walking, the therapist can use the legs to bring the infant's hips forward while facilitating proper trunk righting and rotation as well as diagonal weight shifting with hands on the infant's chest. (Photograph by Carol Herwig.)

and back (Fig. 12). The center of gravity must be aligned with the base of support and the infant must never be allowed to lean or push back. While shifting the weight, the therapist pushes down (diagonally) from the non-weight-bearing shoulder and/or trunk for facilitation of lateral righting. At the same time, this side is slightly rotated backward while the weight-bearing side is slightly rotated forward. The therapist must facilitate the forward weight shift through the weight-bearing side. A common error is to push the pelvis forward on the side where the leg swings forward. This results in internal rotation of both hips and accentuates a frequently abnormal gait pattern. Support is, of course, gradually withdrawn in accordance with the infant's progress.

FACILITATION OF STANDING AND WALKING AS PART OF THE OVERALL PROGRAM

Parents anxiously await the moment when their infant takes the first independent steps. This anxiety is, of course, even greater in parents of a handicapped infant and demands consideration by the therapist. However, there are dangers in pushing an infant toward independence. When the balance for standing and walking takes high priority in the treatment program, the quality of posture may be, to some extent, sacrificed.

Early phases of standing and walking are combined with a broad stance and symmetrical postures. The symmetrical and more primitive postures are, then, also applied in lower positions and the infant seems to regress in postural adjustments. It is, therefore, important not to work exclusively on standing and walking but to continue with some facilitation of mature postural reactions, such as axial rotation and differentiation of motor patterns in other positions that do not threaten the infant's balance.

SUMMARY

The goal of therapy is to provide the infant who demonstrates signs of CNS impairment with the experience of normal patterns of posture and movement. A major concern in all activities is the quality of motor patterns. Special emphasis is placed on proper postural alignment and well-integrated movement patterns of head and shoulder girdle which must be achieved to develop well-coordinated movements throughout the body (Figs. 13a to c).

The program design presented in this chapter focuses on some of the most important motor components and postural subskills of diverse functional activities. Handling techniques have been described in much detail in order to emphasize the importance of correct motor patterns.

It must be stressed that these activities are not applicable to every patient. The samples given must be adapted on an individual basis and the elicited responses must be critically assessed. Furthermore, therapy should offer the infant a vast variety of normal sensorimotor experiences far exceeding the

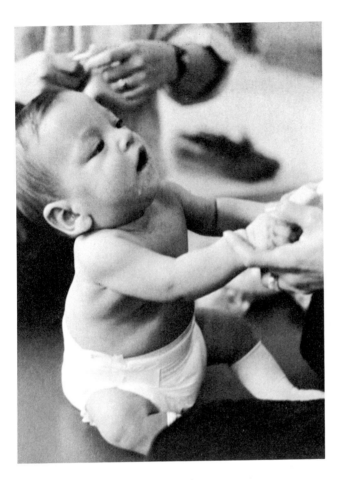

Figure 13a Poor postural control of head, shoulder girdle, and trunk severely restrict this 8-month-old infant in his interaction with the environment and further development in all areas. Compare with Figures 13b and 13c.

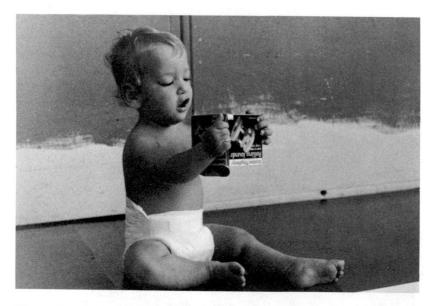

Figure 13b Although his functional skills are not fully age-appropriate after 12 months of treatment, the displayed quality of postural tonus and alignment as well as the variability of his motor patterns indicate good integration of basic postural adjustments. Compare with Figure 13a.

examples given. The observation and analysis of normal motor behavior should serve as a guideline for the design of new activities.

The therapy approach to CNS dysfunction is still in a state of rapid growth and development. This poses exciting challenges to all professionals involved in the treatment of infants who display symptoms of sensorimotor impairment.

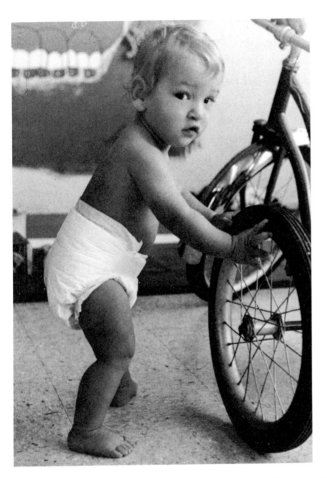

Figure 13c The foundation is laid for taking on the task of learning to master the environment. Compare with Figure 13a.

REFERENCES

1. Jackson, H. J. Selected Writing of John Hughlings Jackson, Vol. 2. (James Taylor, Ed.). London, Staples Press, 1958.

2. Fisher, E. Physiological basis of volitional movements. *Phys. Ther. Rev.* 38:6, 1958.

3. Magnus, R. Körperstellung. Berlin, Springer Verlag, 1924.

4. Schaltenbrand, G. Normale Bewegungs–und Lagereaktionen bei Kindern. *Dtsch. Z. Nerv.* 87:23, 1925.

5. Milani-Comparetti, A., and Gidoni, E. A.: Pattern analysis of motor development and its disorders. *Dev. Med. Child Neurol.* 9:625-630, 1967.

6. Bobath, K., and Bobath, B. The facilitation of normal postural reactions and movements in the treatment of cerebral palsy. *Physiotherapy* 50:246, 1964.

7. Quinton, M. B., and Köng, E. Extensor 1-5, Baby Treatment. Film Kinderklinik, Inselspital, Bern. Maeder Film Limited, Basel, 1977.

BIBLIOGRAPHY

Bobath, B. Treatment principles and planning in cerebral palsy. *Physiotherapy* 49:122, 1963.

Bobath, B. The very early treatment of cerebral palsy. *Dev. Med. Child Neurol* 9:373-390, 1967.

Boehme, R. Improving Upper Body Control. Therapy Skill Builders, Tucson, AZ, 1988.

Forsyth, S. The application of the Bobath philosophy of treatment to the practice of occupational therapy. *South African J Neurodev. Ther* (6)2, September, 1982.

Köng, E. Frühtherapy Zerebraler Bewegungsstörungen. *Med. Welt* 23:446-448, 1972.

Köng, E. Erfahrungen mit der Frühtherapy. *Paediatr. Fortbldg. Praxis* 40: 132-137, 1974.

Smith, M. "Sensory-motor facilitation based on the postural reflex mechanism." In *Selected Proceedings: from Barbro Salek Memorial Symposium*. NDTA, Oak Park, IL, 1984.

Stern, F. M. A Therapist's Contribution to a Follow-up Clinic. In Selected

Proceedings from Barbro Salek Memorial Symposium. NDTA, Oak Park, IL, 1984.

Tauffkirchen, E. Grundzüge der Physiotherapy bei Zerebralparese—nach Bobath. *Paediatr. Praxis* 16:539-549, 1975/76.

Wilson, J. Cerebral palsy. In Campbell, S. (Ed.), Pediatric Neurologic Physical Therapy. Churchill Livingstone, New York, 1984.

9

New Concepts in Therapy

The previous chapters on therapy represent traditional concepts of the neuro-developmental treatment (Bobath) approach. The new clinical insights gained through working with children, sharing ideas with colleagues and students, and, through personal movement experiences in the martial arts seem to be distinctive enough to merit representation as a separate entity in this chapter.

SENSORY AND POSTURAL ORGANIZATION FOR MOVEMENT

Normal and abnormal movement and its developmental processes were discussed in Chapter 4, with emphasis on motor components. The following section accentuates the synthesis of the sensory, motor, and perceptual aspects of movement exemplified in a discussion on the postural reflex mechanism.

Automatic Postural Mechanisms

A major focus in NDT has always been on automatic postural adjustments. The automatic reactions with the strongest effect on the efficiency of volitional and functional movements are postural tonus, reciprocal inhibition, patterns of posture, and movement (i.e., righting and equilibrium reactions), all of which comprise the postural reflex mechanism [1,2].

In this section each component of the postural reflex mechanism is described separately but this must not be construed to mean they develop separately. In addition to the classical definitions, a suggested maturational course and possible additional manifestations of the postural reflex mechanism based on clinical observations are included.

Postural Tonus

Postural tonus describes the muscle tension throughout the body elicited by extero/intero/proprioceptive stimuli. Accordingly, there are three components to consider: (a) degree of stiffness or tension, (b) adaptability, and (c) distribution. Maturation progresses in predictable patterns.

Degree of stiffness. Postural tonus is defined as mature when it is high enough to support the body against gravity yet still low enough to allow for free movements [3]. Observation of babies' postures at various ages suggests that mature organization of tonus is also expressed in the ability to adapt muscle tension in a way that allows optimal contact with the support surface. When contact is optimal, an efficient, active base for the body to support upon and a dynamic base to move from are created. As such this skill becomes the foundation and prerequisite for the criteria upon which tonus is traditionally evaluated (see above definition). Organization of tonus for antigravity posture and movement as well as for an efficient base of support develops in a cephalocaudal direction along the central body axis (see Figs. 1,2,3).

The child with cerebral palsy has difficulties with organizing tonus on that level. Without efficient contact with the support surface, the postural set for antigravity posture and movement is inadequate and therefore the true potential for supporting the body against gravity may not be expressed. Yet, if the examiner provides an efficient base of support through handling, postural tonus in the rest of the body often improves spontaneously. This strategy has proved to be very useful in treatment. By establishing and accentuating an efficient base of support, the therapist enables the infant to posturally organize around it to full potential (see App. Figs. 9-15).

Adaptability. The ability to appropriately adapt tonus according to the ever-changing environmental demands may be functionally even more significant than the absolute strength of tonus. A dynamic stimulus is required to elicit dynamic tonus responses. Such a stimulus may be found in dynamic weight bearing. During early phases of development, each part of the body becomes at one time the base of support upon which the body rights and around which the body moves and orients. In addition to systematically modifying

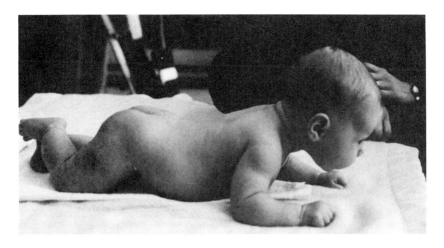

Figure 1 By 3 months of age, babies have sufficient tonus to support the head and upper ribcage against gravity in prone on elbows, but the lower part of the body is not yet posturally organized for an active base of support. An early phase of reciprocal inhibition is expressed in the control of end-range motion of the head. Compare with Figs. 2 and 3.

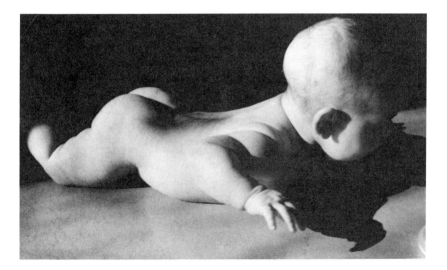

Figure 2 By 4 months, the baby lifts head and upper trunk without support on arms while the lower trunk actively stabilizes into the support surface. Development of reciprocal inhibition has progressed to midrange control of head and neck movements and end-range control of the thoracic spine and the arms. Compare with Figs. 1 and 3.

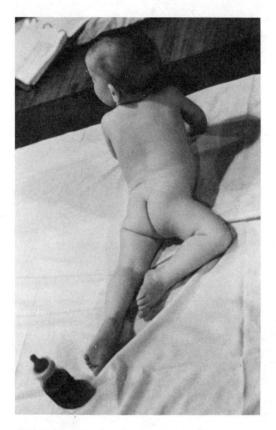

Figure 3 After 6 months of age, babies organize tonus and posture of pelvis and legs to create an efficient base of support for the body to move from. The lumbar spine and hips can be stabilized in end-range of extension allowing midrange control through the rest of the spine. Compare with Figs. 1 and 2.

tonus, this mechanism may also have an important impact on shaping body schema.

In cerebral palsy, abnormal strength and distribution of tonus lead to holding of stereotypic and often static postures resulting in inefficient patterns of weight bearing. The parts of the body that show the most severe hypertonicity never reach full contact with the support surface and fail to receive the

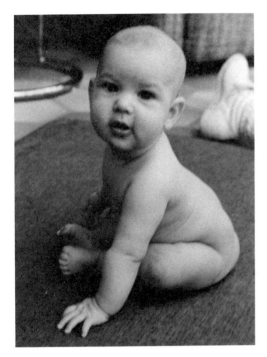

Figure 4 Initial attempts of independent sitting are characterized by low proximal tonus (pelvis and low trunk sink forward) and relatively higher distal tonus (clawing of toes, flexion of fingers). Compare with Fig. 5.

proprioceptive input associated with dynamic pressure. Hypotonicity may allow contact with the supporting surface, but without active contouring and push-off, proprioceptive input is also impoverished. In treatment, dynamic weight bearing drastically changes tonus and fosters the development of a more dynamic, adaptable tonus. In addition, it seems to impact on body schema.

Distribution. Low proximal and relatively higher distal tonus is characteristic for early phases of normal development [4]. Matured tonus is higher proximally, providing proximal stability and lower distally, ensuring maximal distal mobility (see Figs. 4,5).

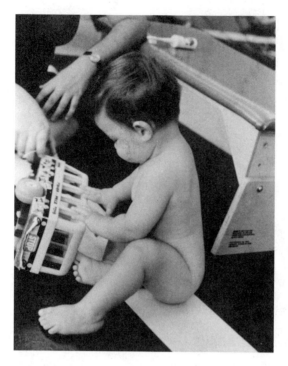

Figure 5 Higher proximal and lower distal tonus provide this 10-month-old baby with dynamic stability of trunk and pelvis, freeing the limbs to move through the full range of motion. Compare with Fig. 4.

In cerebral palsy the discrepancy is more extreme from the onset. The normal reversal of distribution from primitive to mature does not occur. Instead, high compensatory tonus manifests in the limbs, the shoulder girdle, around the hips, in oral areas, and in head and neck muscles while proximal tonus along the spine is often insufficient to support the body against the pull of gravity. Distal compensatory hypertonus (in the body sections described above) is then used for stabilizing and balancing.

For therapy it is suggested not to approach high distal tonus in isolation. Instead, sensory input that organizes tonus along the spine is provided to achieve a spontaneous reduction of high distal tonus and to free the limbs

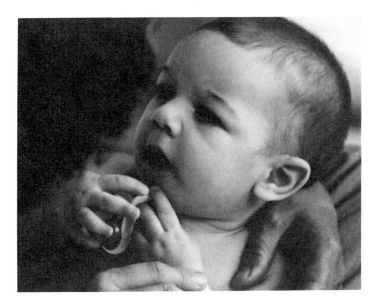

Figure 6 The therapist counteracts excessive tonus and compensatory stability in the fingers with gentle approximation input to wrist and forearm, gradually transferring stability to more proximal parts of the arm (photograph by Phil Koch).

for movement (see App. Figs. 12-15). In a more subtle way one can also channel stability progressively more to proximal body parts with handling. For example, transferring it from the fingers to the wrist by gently loading the wrist for more cocontraction either in space or against a support, then the forearm, etc. (see Fig. 6).

Reciprocal Inhibition

Reciprocal inhibition describes the interplay between agonist (the primary activating muscles) and antagonist (opposing muscles). While the agonist shortens during movement, the antagonist lengthens appropriately. When both agonist and antagonist exert equal force, joints and body parts are stabilized. The importance of reciprocal inhibition for postural control and grading of movement was originally presented by Sherrington (1915). Bobath described the disturbance of reciprocal innervation in cerebral palsy in terms of an excess of cocontraction (i.e., postural stabilization) or an excess of reciprocal inhibition [6].

Maturation of this refined organization seems to emerge at a stage when postural tonus, in specific active movement tonus has matured along the head, neck, and upper trunk, but organization is still primitive throughout the lower part of the body [7]. Reciprocal inhibition matures also in a cephalo to caudal direction.

When fully matured, reciprocal inhibition provides dynamic postural stabilization as well as grading of movement. Stabilization and movement should not be seen as absolutes. In every functional movement there is a portion of the body that is the most stable, versus another part that is the most mobile with the rest of the body showing various gradations in between. Yet, even the most stable part needs to have some mobility and the most mobile part needs to have some stability (true ballistic movements are probably at one end of this scale).

A systematic development of postural stabilization and grading of movement is suggested. First, control is established in end ranges of motion and last in midranges. This process can be followed section by section throughout the body in a cephalo to caudal direction (see Figs. 1,2,3).

In cerebral palsy reciprocal innervation is poorly coordinated. The balance between postural stabilization and movement is disturbed. Stabilization may be excessive and static and is often found only in end ranges. Movements, on the other hand, may lack sufficient stability and grading.

To apply the above observations to treatment means to look for the systematic achievement of static, then dynamic stability, first in end ranges and then in midranges and also to work for it in the right sequence throughout the body. For example, unless the low lumbar spine develops control in the full end range of extension, compensatory and excessive extension has to be used through the thoracic and upper lumbar spine in many positions, and therefore, dynamic midrange control is not developed (see App. Figs. 14,15).

As to the exact stimulus provided by the therapist, it should always be directed toward the agonist for shortening and toward the antagonist for simultaneous lengthening. For the delicate balance between opposing muscle groups this method of handling seems to be better suited than activating only on one side of the joint (for a more detailed description see later section on Kinesthetic Input).

Patterns of Posture and Movement

The various righting and equilibrium reactions are the automatic motor patterns most important for efficiency of movement.

RIGHTING REACTIONS

Righting reactions enable babies in every position to properly orient the head in space, that is, with the face in the vertical and the eyes in the horizontal plane and to achieve the most efficient body alignment around and along three body axes. This specific head orientation and body alignment have been defined by Magnus in animal experiments [8] as righting reactions. Schaltenbrand described the systematic development of various righting reactions in the human infant [9]. Bobath relates these observations to patients with cerebral palsy [10].

Many clinicians use the term for postures and movements against gravity even when the criteria of the definition are not met. This leads to substantial miscommunication since righting reactions represent a certain degree of sensory, perceptual, and motor organization and are therefore indicative of a certain level of CNS maturation. Skill level and prognosis differ greatly for the infant who moves without such a degree of organization.

The righting reactions develop over the first months of life, with the exception of neck righting which is present at birth and realigns body and head whenever the head is substantially rotated to the side, backward, or forward. Even though the other righting reactions are not present at birth or at best are immature, newborns and young infants can momentarily align the head when held upright with proper support through the trunk. They seem to "know" where the proper alignment is but lack sufficient motor control. Patients with central nervous system (CNS) dysfunction seem "not to know" how to align and orient. Babies can and do move against gravity without mature righting reactions since movement against gravity occurs as a function of postural tonus, it is the proper head orientation and body alignment which are functions of the righting reactions. Most of the righting reactions become integrated into equilibrium reactions.

Head posture and body alignment (i.e., proper righting) have always been an important focus in neurodevelopmental treatment and corrective/supportive input has been applied in various ways to achieve this. Instead of correcting the motor output, as is done traditionally, previously described concepts can be applied here: create the correct tactile and proprioceptive stimuli that elicit the respective righting reactions by establishing exact weight-bearing patterns. Accentuated loading of the system is often necessary and can be achieved by additional pressure input. By focusing on organizing the sensory input preceding the motor response, the therapist's input follows a direction different from that of the elicited motor response (see Kinesthetic Input).

EQUILIBRIUM REACTIONS

Just as righting reactions define very specific postures against gravity so are equilibrium reactions only one—the most efficient—means of balancing. Equilibrium reactions are automatic and are the only balance reactions that fully incorporate righting reactions, that is, proper spatial orientation of the head and the most efficient postural alignment. Patterns of equilibrium reactions have been described by Weisz [11], Rademaker [12], and Zador [13]. Bobath investigates equilibrium reactions in normal and handicapped children [3,6,10].

As with righting reactions, the term is often applied regardless of quality and form of the motor pattern. Yet babies are able to balance before equilibrium reactions are matured using a variety of balancing strategies, such as, (a) a broad base of support, and (b) compensatory postures and exaggerated postural stabilization in one part of the body to compensate for lack of dynamic stability in another part of the body. "High guard" posturing is such a compensation. Excessive distal stabilization is another compensation for lack of proximal stability.

Equilibrium reactions maintain the most efficient relationship of the center of gravity to the base of support during any movement or when the whole body is in motion or when the support surface moves. This can be achieved in two ways: by aligning the center of gravity over the base of support, the classical equilibrium reaction, or by bringing the base of support under the center of gravity. Both ways require a keen kinesthetic awareness of this relationship.

For the most part, therapists concentrate on the first option, (the classical equilibrium reaction). This reaction is elicited either by moving the infant on a stable support, or by placing the child on a movable equipment, such as a ball or roll and moving the equipment (the support). Clinical experience indicates it may be easier to establish a sense of balanced alignment by encouraging first adaptations of the base of support to proximal weight shifts as they occur, for example, during transitions (see App. Fig. 20).

Also, the concept of maintaining or returning the center of gravity over the base of support is developed with small excursions of weight shift, such as during such activities as looking back over the shoulder, lifting one leg to pull the sock over the heel, reaching for objects that are positioned beyond arm's length. For that reason ambitious ball activities often result in some improvement of compensatory balancing skills instead of eliciting true equilibrium reactions.

Instead of focusing on the *specific patterns* of equilibrium reactions it seems more helpful to attend to more *general concepts of postural organization* underlying the whole range of equilibrium reactions. The three most important concepts are: (1) to weight shift through the lower part of the body (low trunk, pelvis, legs) (see App. Fig. 24). This permits head and trunk to be brought into proper alignment (as a function of righting and equilibrium). (2) To actively stabilize the base of support so that the center of gravity can be moved over it. This requires a high degree of dissociation; for example, to activate into one direction for stability (into the base of support) and to activate simultaneously into another direction for movement (see Figs. 7,8). (3) To adapt the posture of the limbs to proximal weight shifts (see App. Figs. 13,20). Progress in these three areas will significantly improve the efficiency of balancing.

INTEGRATION

The individual components of the postural reflex mechanism do not develop in isolation nor in unison. There is an overlapping sequencing in their development [7]: active movement tonus develops first in a cephalo to caudal direction. This follows the caudo to cephalic development of other aspects of tonus which starts in utero [4]. Before organization of tonus has fully matured throughout the body, maturation of reciprocal inhibition emerges starting at head and neck. Next, righting reactions develop, and lastly equilibrium reactions which require that all other components have matured. Before completion of this process, babies show maturity and competence in some parts of the body and simultaneously primitive patterns in other sections.

In cerebral palsy this interweaving pattern of development does not happen. Attempts to move against gravity result in progressively more abnormal or compensatory tonus throughout the body, while postures of head, neck, and upper trunk indicate that maturation of reciprocal innervation or righting has not begun [7]. The postural patterns deviate from the norm at every developmental stage; they are inefficient and perpetuate more pathology.

TREATMENT GOALS

By introducing ways to elicit and shape reactions of the postural reflex mechanism Bobath [14] has addressed the automatic aspect of movement which is always disturbed in cerebral palsy. Selectively eliciting automatic

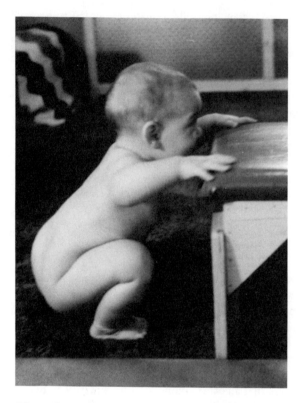

Figure 7   The ability to actively stabilize the legs down into the support makes possible forward movement of pelvis and trunk over that base. Activation with such a degree of dissociation is an important aspect of equilibrium reactions. Compare with Fig. 8.

responses through handling makes it possible to treat babies with movement disorders [3,15] . The original assumption was that patients will spontaneously integrate into volitional and functional activities the automatic responses evoked in therapy. It was later realized that many children needed help with integrating new postural adaptations into functional activities. Yet the early concepts influenced many therapists and led to a distorted view regarding the degree to which function depends on a mature postural reflex mechanism and treatment goals were often set for "normalizing" tonus, developing righting

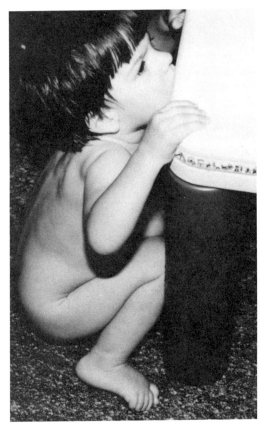

Figure 8 A highly associated pull into flexion interferes with actively stabilizing the legs against the support. This toddler relies for balancing on the
tight grip with both hands. Compare with Fig. 7.

and equilibrium reactions, and so on, without specific reference to function.
Besides these global postural milestones, a very narrow focus on specific
movement components, such as scapular adduction and abdominal control
seem to be equally remote from functional activities that are meaningful to
child and parent. Also, attempts to facilitate mature, if not perfect, postural
responses gave scant attention to the patient's sensory limitations in coping

with a drastic change of motor patterns. The concern with long-term effects
of abnormal motor patterns misled some therapists to prevent a child from
performing a function if it only could be carried out abnormally (for example, W sitting) instead of trying to counteract the negative effects on the mus-
culoskeletal system during activities performed in other positions.

In response, functional training with little regard to quality of movement
was promoted by some clinicians. Such an approach can improve the skill
level in functional activities and developmental milestones even when the postural organization does not improve. These children learn to make better use
of abnormal movement patterns, which in the process of excessive use become increasingly more predominant and habitual. However, the success may
be short-term because postural compensations that are sufficient for simple
activities become increasingly less efficient for higher and more demanding
functions.

In recent years the Bobaths have repeatedly stressed that function must be
the primary treatment goal in NDT without neglecting the role automatic
postural mechanisms play in regard to the efficiency of function.

Function and Essential Postural Organization

A holistic approach to motor dysfunction may be realized by combining
functional activities as the treatment goal with the underlying postural organization as the postural objective or means to reach this functional goal.
The treatment goal should be child and family oriented, consisting of a clearly defined function that impacts on the child's present situation. Therapists
then use their expertise in movement and motor development to select as
secondary goals or postural objectives those aspects of postural organization
that are most important for the respective function and for the next stage of
development. By selecting only certain aspects of righting, equilibrium,
organization of tonus, or reciprocal innervation instead of aiming for the
completely mature pattern, the postural goals become attainable.

Function may be easily described once infants have developed sufficient
physical independence to transform their intentions into actions. It is more
difficult to delineate realistic functional goals for the mentally retarded child
and not to sacrifice function for pure form [16]. Designing functional goals
for infants, specifically during the early stages of development, challenges
us to a broader view of the infant's competencies, acknowledging that motor
skills are prepared by and, conversely, impact on sensory, perceptual, social,
and emotional skills. "Soft neurological signs" indicate that the inability to
organize is not restricted to motor behavior alone, but may find expression

in any function. For treatment it means being alert to improvement in everyday activities in association with better sensory and postural organization; the mere improvement of a motor response to a stimulus is not sufficient.

A few examples of early as well as more mature functions (*treatment goals*) and underlying postural organization (*postural objectives*) are described below.

1. One early functional competence that may be affected by CNS dysfunction is the ability to adapt to and cope with stimuli of everyday activities. Caretaking activities provide a multitude of tactile, proprioceptive, and kinesthetic input. Normally, responsiveness to these stimuli is exceptionally high during early months of life and represents an important avenue of learning. Habituation to stimuli of routine activities enables infants to attend to and learn from novel situations, sights, and sounds. Irritable behavior or hypertonic posturing often are elicited by regular tactile, proprioceptive, and kinesthetic input in infants with CNS dysfunction.

While the functional goal may lie in successful management of dressing, feeding, carrying, etc., the postural objective is in the area of adaptation to touch, pressure, and movements associated with the respective activity. A systematic and sensitive approach is necessary regarding location, amount, and duration of touch or pressure, and also regarding direction and speed of movement. The initial input is very gentle and only gradually increased according to the infant's acceptance. The infant is not expected to "do" anything, yet adapting to these inputs is nevertheless an active response (a function of organization of tonus). The parent needs to be advised on optimally matching some of the handling inputs to the routine activities of caretaking.

2. Orientation to visual and auditory stimuli is another early function that is present even before righting reactions are fully matured. Posturally, this requires that much of the weight be shifted down to the low trunk while in prone or supine, so that the head is free to move. Excitement and effort may lead to a burst of uncoordinated movements which interferes with balance and must be counteracted with some stabilizing into the support.

For more mature head righting as needed for visual tracking and monitoring or reach in prone, the posture of pelvis and legs must be adapted to create an efficient and gradually more active base of support (see App. Figs. 9-15).

3. Self-calming by sucking on the hand may be difficult for the infant with poor postural organization. The hands may be used for distal stabilization leading to compensatory high tonus. In addition to activating the infant more proximally for stability, the therapist may have to work more directly on adaptation of tonus through the upper extremity as well as in the

oral area. Deep pressure to face or upper extremity simulate weight bearing and superimposed, gentle movements simulate weight shifting. Both are excellent means for modification of tonus and can be carried out in a variety of positions.

4. Exploring body and environment visually and manually is an important input for the development of body schema and perceptual competencies. Mouthing of hands, feet, and objects brings another dimension to this investigation. Posturally, the infant needs to stabilize proximally so that shoulder girdle and arms can move on the trunk to reach or for legs and feet to be brought toward the hands or the mouth while in supine (see App. Fig. 11).

5. Holding and releasing objects while reaching are difficult functions for the posturally insecure infant. Establishing some degree of proximal (i.e., spinal) stability may again be one postural objective. Another objective is the ability to contour the hand to objects of various sizes, firmness, and texture. Initially this is achieved by "weight bearing" into these objects, although not with a flat hand usually associated with weight bearing, but in a grasping posture around the object being held. The same can be achieved with the hand contoured to various body parts. The therapist cradles the infant's hand and provides equal pressure in all directions in order not to flatten the infant's hand. Gradually the therapist's proprioceptive cuing and feedback are reduced so that a more discriminatory touch can develop.

6. The ability to change positions allows infants to maneuver themselves in relation to desirable objects and to see their surroundings from various angles. For efficient and controlled transitions postural adaptations must occur throughout the body: proximal weight shift is accompanied by adapting the posture of the limbs for support. Many handicapped children use excessive head movements for shifting weight and maintain a static, inactive leg posture (see App. Figs. 12-15). Proper positioning and stabilizing of the legs support weight shifts, freeing the arms for manipulative skills and providing balance for transitions.

7. Reaching and manipulation are often difficult or impossible when the shoulder girdle is used for compensatory (distal) postural stability. Improving shoulder girdle mobility as the postural objective can only be achieved if the postural stability is transferred to the spine. Proximal weight shift through low trunk and pelvis is another postural objective during dynamic play activities (see App. Fig. 24) or when raising the infant's leg during dressing or pushing an arm through a sleeve, etc.

8. A means of progression affords the child a large degree of independence, specifically, ambulation which is often though a very long-term goal.

For any form of progression a necessary postural skill lies in actively stabilizing the legs as a base of support while moving pelvis and trunk over that base. A prerequisite of that skill is the ability to create an efficient and dynamic base of support in the position used for progression. Some suggestions on how to prepare feet for standing and walking were made in Chapter 8. Balance reactions of legs and feet can also be prepared through weight bearing in prone, supine, various sitting postures, and during transitions (see Figs. 11, 18-23). Providing accentuated pressure input to lower legs and feet while crawling heightens the awareness of a dynamic base of support (see Fig. 22).

9. Although a parent's goal of ambulation should always be respected, some other goals may have to be interjected as shorter term, such as improving balance in supported standing. This can be applied to play activities with the child standing at a coffee table or sofa. Balance can only be achieved when the center of gravity (low trunk and pelvis) can be aligned over the base of support (feet). This aspect of righting and equilibrium may be difficult not only on a motor but also sensory and perceptual levels. Strong sensory reinforcement given through the therapist's handling accentuates awareness and feedback. The proper alignment always decreases spasticity in the legs and may even result in a lack of support tonus. To create more tonus the therapist may have to bombard the system with prolonged and heavy (but global) weight-bearing pressure.

10. Vocalizing and sound play can be compromised by compensatory postural stabilization in the oral and pharyngeal area. As a postural objective, an efficient base of support must be established with input for stability through spine, pelvis and legs (see App. Figs. 16,17). Weight shifting may also have to be channeled caudally to pelvis and low trunk (see App. Figs. 18-22). During balance activities it is important not to challenge the infant to the point where these compensations, which are not readily visible, occur.

11. Pitch and volume of voice cannot be modulated when spine and pelvis lack dynamic stability as a base for graded movements of the ribcage. Postural organization needs to occur in a cephalo to caudal direction along the spine, pelvis and legs. The body weight must be directed caudally down into the base of support. This contrasts with abnormal, where placement of body weight and compensatory counterbalancing occurs to a large degree in the anterior/posterior direction (see App. Figs. 16, 17).

While the above examples are given in more general terms, it is suggested for the individual case to more accurately specify the functional goals and the postural objectives as to sensory input provided, the expected response and the position(s) used.

HANDLING

General principles of handling have been described in Chapter 8. Now, handling input is related specifically, to those concepts of sensory and postural organization that have been discussed in this chapter. Handling is used to organize sensory stimuli for the patient. Tactile, proprioceptive, and kinesthetic input must be coordinated with the activity and must be adapted to the needs of each patient. The therapist prepares movement by providing selective tactile and proprioceptive input *before* giving any movement cue.

Tactile Input

The initial touch sets the stage for the infant's reaction to being handled; the more global it is, the more organizing it is. Therapists need to adapt tonus in their own hands to achieve maximal contouring to the infant's body and to equally distribute the contact. This leads to the initial handling input being subthreshold to achieve accommodation before stronger and more directive stimuli are used.

Proprioceptive Input

Once adaptation to the tactile stimulus has been accomplished, pressure is used to add proprioceptive input. If the force used by the therapist is generated proximally rather than from arms or hands it is less stressful and less likely to create tension in the therapist's hands. When tension is present, it is always translated to the patient. A gradual buildup of force helps to elicit an efficient recruiting pattern in both the therapist and the patient. How therapists align their own center of gravity relative to their hands determines the amount of pressure input.

Kinesthetic Input

The directionality of pressure adds to kinesthetic input. Accuracy is important, otherwise joints may be exposed to shearing forces. The direction of movement and of cocontraction is always three dimensional. Movement is traditionally described as flexion, extension, lateral flexion, and rotation; but this describes only the rotations around the three body axes. In addition, translations occur along each axis, that is, a sliding motion in the anterior-posterior, side to side, and cephalocaudal directions. In functional movements the common pathway of the various rotations and translations describes an arc in the configuration of a helix [17] or various sections thereof, the concave and convex sides representing the shortening and lengthening on opposite sides of joints. The direction of the therapist's input can therefore never be in straight or diagonal lines. The pressure input always describes a three-dimensional arc crossing the axes of joints in order to grade activation on both sides for well-organized reciprocal innervation.

Proprioceptive and kinesthetic input are, furthermore, directed into the base of support, that is, in a direction different from the direction of movement that occurs off and around that base. An example can be seen in Fig. 17. For better sitting posture, the therapist's input to the lumbar spine is directed toward the upper thighs and sitting bones crossing the horizontal and vertical body axes; it is convex to the front to elongate the flexors and concave to the back to shorten the extensors of the trunk.

SUMMARY

By stressing the importance of the postural reflex mechanism for efficiency of functional activities the therapy approach described in this chapter incorporates neurodevelopmental treatment (NDT) concepts. The relationship between function and postural automatic mechanisms is investigated via a few examples applicable to infants. Emphasis is on the importance of selecting functional treatment goals while the underlying postural organization is seen as an objective or means to achieve these functions.

The described interpretation regarding possible manifestations and developmental processes of the postural reflex mechanism led to treatment procedures that differ in certain aspects from the traditional practice of NDT. These treatment procedures and their underlying rationale derived from concepts which were established in 1943 by the Bobaths and which have since been enriched and refined by lessons learned from patients. The following points attempt to delineate traditional NDT concepts from the approach described in this chapter.

In general terms, the emphasis on motor patterns per se is less pronounced than traditionally occurs; instead, the focus on kinesthetic perception and sensory cues surrounding and preceding motor patterns takes priority.

1. Good postural alignment and positional control are seen as secondary to the ability to create an efficient base of support. If tonus cannot be adapted at the base, it will be poorly organized throughout; similarly, the tactile and proprioceptive stimuli that elicit righting reactions also require certain weight-bearing patterns. The ability to use the arms freely for manipulation can only develop when pelvis and legs take on the task of forming a

dynamic base of support in all positions. In treatment, attention shifts from patterns of movement to patterns of weight bearing and to the efficiency of the base of support. Contouring to the support surface and dynamic weight bearing are elicited through global tactile, proprioceptive, and kinesthetic input.

2. Regarding tonus problems, the emphasis is transferred to distribution and adaptability. Working on either or both changes the degree of stiffness. Adaptability of tonus must first be achieved relative to the support surface before tonus can be adapted to postures and movements in space. The support surface can be a piece of equipment, the infant's body (e.g., hands for weight bearing on the mouth), or the therapist's body or hands. For dynamic weight bearing, small weight shifts are imposed while assisting the infant with optimal contouring and necessary postural adaptations at the base. For example, in sitting, a lateral weight shift is combined with a small increase of abduction and external rotation in both legs. Traditionally, hypertonus is modified by changing alignment and/or orientation in space; reducing effort; moving the child through certain patterns; using specific, localized handling techniques, such as tapping to increase tonus.

Based on the discussion in the first section of this chapter, areas of hypertonicity often are interpreted to be an expression of compensatory postural stability. Through proprioceptive, kinesthetic input the therapist distributes stability more appropriately throughout the body to achieve optimal motility where needed.

3. Instead of eliciting the classical equilibrium reactions, this approach tries to foster more fundamental movement percepts of the relationship between center of gravity and base of support, such as (a) bringing the base of support under the center of gravity, (b) establishing a weight shift through pelvis and legs, and (c) activating into the base of support for stability in one part of the body while activating off that base (in a different direction) for movement. During one treatment session, the therapist may work on only one of these skills but does so in a variety of positions. Strong proprioceptive input is used to heighten the awareness of how the center of gravity relates to the base of support.

4. Patterns of posture and movement are described as occurring in end range or midrange rather than, for example, in flexion or extension. The infant is expected to achieve control in both end ranges before grading movements in mid ranges. This means therapists don't pursue a change from abnormal to mature movement patterns, but "detour" first to early and less

efficient movement patterns modeling after sequencing in normal development.

5. Postural support provided through handling or through adaptive equipment is assessed not only as to its postural effectiveness, but also as to the sensory messages signaled to the infant, for example, where to seek stability, where the pivoting point for movement is, where to push off from, where to lean into, etc. Abnormal distribution of tonus or sensorily alignment may be reinforced by corrective support that seems to work biomechanically.

6. Traditionally, therapists describe six degrees of freedom of movement (i.e., rotations) around the three body axes. By adding translations along each axis that number increases to 12, and consequently changes the direction of each functional movement or force of postural stabilizatio.1 to a three-dimensional, helical arc [17].

7. A further difference lies in the direction of therapeutic input. Traditionally, NDT therapists handle from keypoints of control to either stabilize or to guide movements; to facilitate or inhibit the motor output and through it make the child's reactions as normal as possible.

According to the concepts presented in this chapter, the therapist tries to modify tonus, alignment, and movement patterns more indirectly, for example, by accentuating weight bearing input into the base of support (i.e., into gravity) around which the body must orient. The direction of this "weight bearing force" changes constantly during movement. Also, handling is never used to either stimulate the agonist or to inhibit the antagonist. Instead, the therapist always tries to simultaneously effect both, agonist and antagonist by directing the input such that it crosses the axes of joints in an arc.

Contrary to traditional handling, the cues are often given in a direction different from the direction of movement. Well-adapted tactile, proprioceptive, and kinesthetic input is used to load the system in a certain way, waiting for the infant to posturally organize around this global stimulus and to move when ready.

APPENDIX

The following photo sequences exemplify concepts on organizing tactile, proprioceptive, and kinesthetic input given by the therapist to improve efficiency of posture and movement. For more in-depth information please see text.

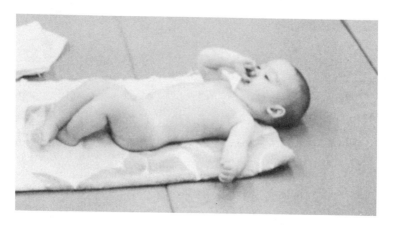

Figure 9 Compensatory distal tonus through the lower extremities has become so strong a habit pattern that it is used even in this well-supported position. High tonus is expressed in hands and feet. The same posture can be seen in Figs. 12 and 14 (photograph by Sherry Arndt).

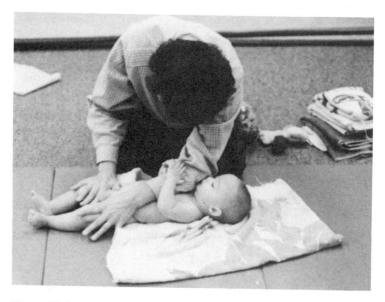

Figure 10 The therapist provides proprioceptive input in the direction of extension, external rotation, abduction of the hips combined with a slight caudal weight shift. Pressure is gradually increased, waiting for the infant to adapt to the weight-bearing pressure and to actively change posture and tonus accordingly. In response, the hands have opened spontaneously and the feet relax. Compare with Fig. 9 (photograph by Sherry Arndt).

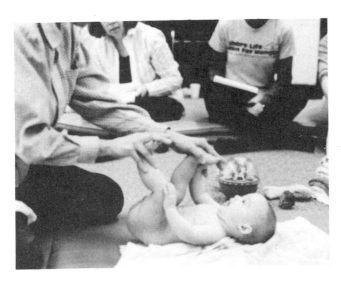

Figure 11 After achieving a more mature distribution of tonus, the legs can be raised for manual and visual exploration. The therapist directs a weight-bearing force through the legs toward the pelvis to stabilize it against the support to allow the legs to move on a stable proximal base (photograph by Sherry Arndt).

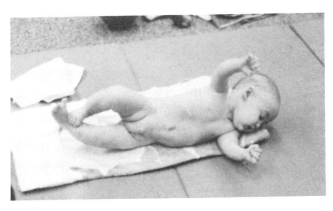

Figure 12 With the limbs pulled off the support this baby has a poor base upon which to right head and upper trunk during rolling. The effort occasioned by the inefficiency of this pattern increases the distal hypertonicity while the trunk remains inactive. Compare with Fig. 13 (photograph by Sherry Arndt).

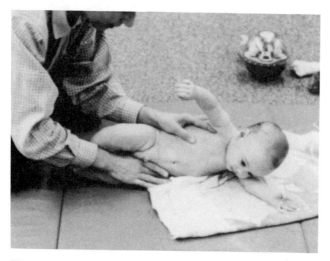

Figure 13 The therapist directs her input toward weight-bearing through lower trunk, pelvis, and leg. The resulting base of support and proximal stability unveil the infant's competence for head righting and spontaneous placement of the right arm and leg to support the proximal weight shift. Compare with Fig. 12 (photograph by Sherry Arndt).

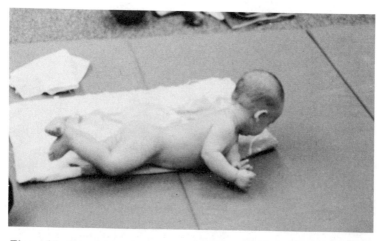

Figure 14 To achieve the necessary weight shift for rolling, this infant uses excessive head motion to compensate for the relative inactivity of the trunk. With greater weight on the thorax, the arms cannot be moved for efficient placement. Compare with Fig. 15 (photography by Sherry Arndt).

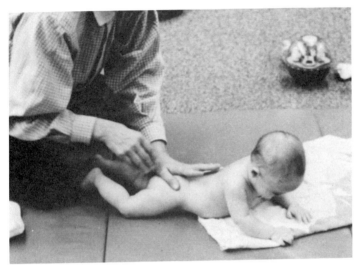

Figure 15 Assisted by the therapist's input, the baby is able to create an active and efficient base of support through lower trunk, pelvis, and legs, freeing the upper part of the body to move. The hips and lumbar spine move toward end range of extension, making possible midrange alignment through thoracic spine, head, and neck. Compare with Fig. 14 (photograph by Sherry Arndt).

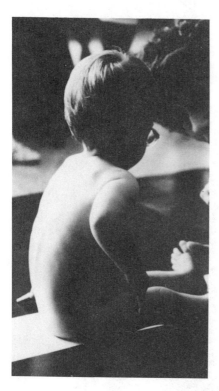

Figure 16 Low proximal stability is compensated by hypertonic distal posturing in the end range of motion (feet in eversion, shoulder girdle pulled forward). This pattern is habitually used in all positions (see Fig. 21). The child lets much of the body weight sink backward into the flexed low thorax and counterbalances by bringing head and upper trunk forward. This can lead to compensatory tightness in oral and pharyngeal areas. Compare with Fig. 17 (photograph by Carol Sussi).

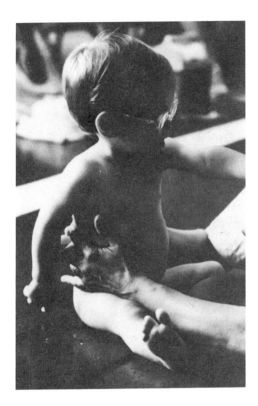

Figure 17 To achieve better cephalocaudal organization along the spine, the therapist's input is directed downward and forward. By accentuating active weight bearing, antigravity tonus and stability are generated throughout the spine. The pressure input on the thigh is from above only so as not to stimulate adduction against the therapist's arm, a compensatory pattern frequently used by the motor handicapped child. Compare with Fig. 16 (photograph by Carol Sussi).

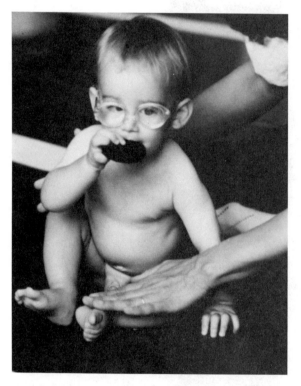

Figure 18   Dynamic adaptation of lower extremity posture in response to proximal weight shift may be an unfamiliar movement concept for the infant who habitually uses the legs for compensatory static stability. The therapist's input aims for optimal contouring of the legs to the support surface and accentuates the proprioceptive feedback (photograph by Carol Sussi).

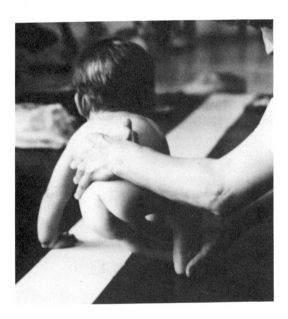

Figure 19 When better distribution of tonus and proximal stability are achieved, more challenging equilibrium responses can be elicited with the whole body orienting dynamically around a distal base of support. The right foot is actively stabilized with assistance in a well-aligned posture. Compare with Figs. 16 and 21 (photography by Carol Sussi).

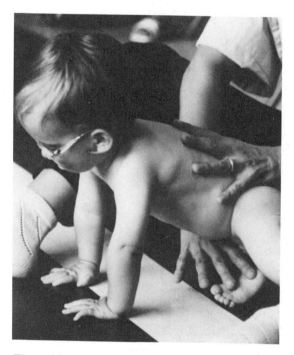

Figure 20 By outwardly rotating the right leg, the infant prepares an efficient base of support for the transition from quadruped to sitting. Throughout the whole movement sequence the therapist monitors adaptation of tonus
and posture of the lower extremities (see Figs. 18 and 19) to counteract a
habitual compensatory pattern as seen in Fig. 21. The input from trunk and
pelvis is directed at the changing base of support as a stimulus for proximal
weightshift and movement (photograph by Carol Sussi).

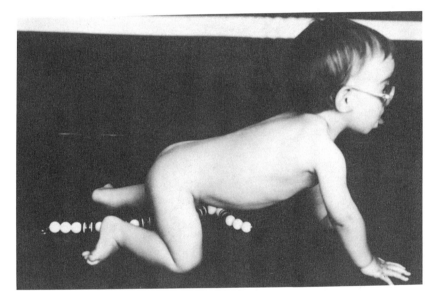

Figure 21   Static stability is achieved in this position through distal high tonus, including the oral area and the feet. The wide base of support makes weight shifting very difficult. Compare with Figs. 22 and 23 (photography by Carol Sussi).

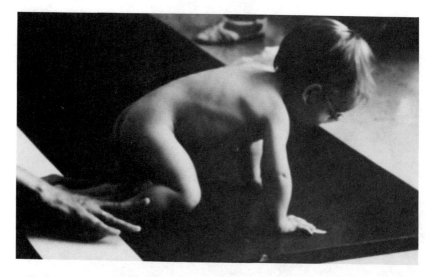

Figure 22   The therapist's proprioceptive input ensures a more efficient and more dynamic base of support during crawling. Contact with the support is maintained also in the foot of the progressing leg which moves forward in a half circle (convex to the midline of the body) to yield external rotation and abduction of the hip and rotation of pelvis and spine. Compare with Fig. 21 (photograph by Carol Sussi).

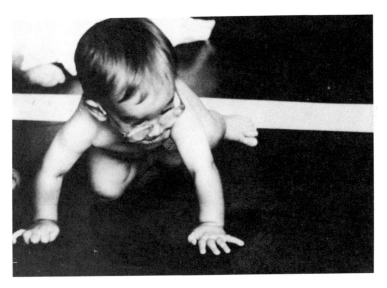

Figure 23 With more proximal stability the need for excessive distal tonus and posturing is negated and a spontaneous weight shift is achieved with the pelvis and trunk rotating against a stable shoulder girdle. Compare with Fig. 21 (photograph by Carol Sussi).

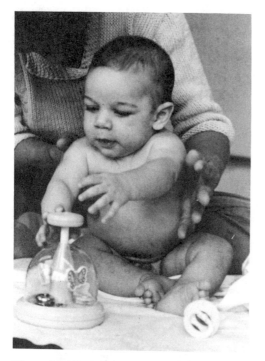

Figure 24 Through deep proprioceptive input directed toward the spine, the therapist transfers postural stabilization from the shoulder girdle (compensatory) to the spine (proximal). Reaching requires for the shoulder girdle to move on a stable spine and for trunk and pelvis to move in the direction of reach. Input for weight shift through lower trunk, pelvis, and legs is superimposed on the therapist's proprioceptive input through her own weight shift (photograph by Phil Koch).

REFERENCES

1. Bobath, K. The normal postural reflex mechanism and its deviation in children with cerebral palsy. *Physiotherapy* 57:515-525, 1971.

2. Bobath, K. A neurophysiological basis for the treatment of cerebral palsy. *Clin. Dev. Med.* 75, Lippincott, Philadelphia, 1980.

3. Bobath, K., and Bobath, B. The facilitation of normal postural reactions and movements in the treatment of cerebral palsy. *Physiotherapy* 50: 245-262, 1964.

4. Saint-Anne Dargassies, S. Neurological Development in the Full-Term and Premature Neonate. Elsevier, Amsterdam, 1977.

5. Sherrington, CS: Reflex inhibition as a factor in the co-ordination of movements and postures. *Quart. J. Exp. Physiol.* 6:251, 1913.

6. Bobath, K. Motor deficit in patients with cerebral palsy. *Clin. Dev. Med.* 23, Heinemann, London, 1966.

7. Tscharnuter, I. The Postural Reflex Mechanism. In Selected Proceedings From the Barbro Salek Memorial Symposium. Neuro-Developmental Treatment Association, Inc., Oak Park, IL, 1984.

8. Magnus, R: Körperstellung. Springer Verlag, Berlin, 1924.

9. Schaltenbrand, G. Normale Bewegungs - und Lagereaktionen bei Kinolern. *Dtch. Z. Nervenheilk.* 87:23, 1925.

10. Bobath, B. Abnormal Postural Reflex Activity Caused by Brain Lesions. Heinemann, London, 1965.

11. Weisz, St. Studies in equilibrium reactions. *J. Nerv. Ment. Dis.* 88:150-162, 1938.

12. Rademaker, G. C. J. Réactions Labyrinthiques et Equilibre. Masson, Paris, 1935.

13. Zador, J. Les Réactions d'Equilibre chez l'Homme. Masson, Paris, 1938.

14. Bobath, B. A new treatment of lesions of the upper motor neuron. *Brit. J. Phys. Med.* 11:26-29, 1948.

15. Bobath, B. The very early treatment of cerebral palsy. *Dev. Med. Child Neurol.* 9:373-390, 1967.

16 Campbell, P. H., and Bricker, W. A. Programming for the severely handicapped person. In J. Gardner, L. Long, R. Nichols, and D. Iagulli (Eds.), Program Issues in Developmental Disabilities. Paul H. Brookes Publishers, Baltimore, 1980.

17. Levin, St. M. The Icosahedron as the Three-Dimensional Finite Element in Biomechanical Support. A Natural Hierarchical System. Lecture presented at Michigan State University, College of Osteopathic Medicine. Dec. 16, 1986. Author's Address: Potomac Back Center, 5021 Seminary Road, Alexandria, Virginia 22311.

10

Assessment of the Management–Treatment Program

CONCEPT OF TREATMENT ASSESSMENT

Traditionally, clinical appraisal of the results of *surgical* treatment in cerebral palsy patients has been a well-established procedure [1]. Many of the evaluations emphasized case reports and utilized follow-up studies. Up to the present, the approach has been similar, although reviews of sizable samples are now more commonly employed [2] than simply individual case studies.

Effectiveness studies of nonsurgical and particularly multispecialty treatment approaches generally are a more recent development. The concept of formal therapy resulting in definitive change has been slow in developing. Rather, a variety of intuitive methods were applied almost more as a humanistic or supportive endeavor than a distinctive form of treatment. The approach to therapy detailed in Chapters 7 and 8 is the culmination and synthesis of advancement in theory and clinical practice to date. Its design for the individual patient today and its future applicability both rest on objective assessment procedures which attempt to identify the influence of the treatment procedure itself in effecting developmental change. It is clear that many variables may play a part in the process of neurological growth and maturation. Confirming the definitive role of a therapy program in affecting this process presents a major challenge to those whose clinical experience is devoted to this effort.

Two major issues are identified: (a) is the individual treatment program effective and appropriate for the given child? (b) is the treatment procedure substantiated by a body of data that includes long-term results? Evaluation of an individual treatment program must be based upon the following: (a) baseline developmental status of the child; (b) a total plan of care into which therapy is integrated; (c) management goals, and (d) treatment goals.

Individual treatment of the child should not be a separate and isolated procedure. It must realistically address the special needs identified in the evaluation; therapy should take its place among a variety of approaches which may include counseling and direction of parents, specialized design of physical features of the home as necessary, among many other possibilities. Most important, both short- and long-range goals developed must realistically relate to the needs of the child and the outlook for his or her future function. Goals for management and facilitation of child care must be considered equally with treatment objectives that may influence neurological change.

A procedure of regular assessment should therefore be part of the individual treatment regime. At periodic intervals it is essential to review changes in management problems, socialization, neurological status, and functional ability in relation to objectives. Interviews with parents and other professionals can be used effectively to update documentation of management and social maturity. This could be further supplemented by psychological testing using such instruments as the Vineland Social Maturity Scale [3]. Clinical therapy evaluation of the infant should include assessment of tone, reflex behavior, developmental patterns of head and neck control, trunk stability, sitting, standing, use of extremities and walking, oral development, hand use, and perceptual ability. A specific format for reevaluation should be utilized to ensure uniformity and completeness. An example of such a form in use is given in the Appendix.

On the basis of the clinical appraisal, judgment will be made to either continue or modify the treatment program, or its relationship to other influencing factors. Many intangibles must be considered including travel to the therapy site, the physical environment, and personality and relationship with the therapist. Any or all of these features or others may influence change and have an effect on outcome. The clinician must be in as objective a position as possible to decide whether a given program is adequately reaching the defined goals and when a change in emphasis or approach is indicated. The process of regular review needs to be included from the beginning in the procedure of working with the child.

The larger issue of long-term effectiveness of a given therapy procedure or approach and development of more effective methods continues to be an urgent professional need. As indicated in Chapter 3, several modalities are in current use. The general clinical impression from available studies using varying test instruments and designs is that early intervention is clearly related to neurological change in early follow-up [4-6]. However, data are totally lacking on the superiority of one method over another or of long-term effects. In more than 30 years of intensive therapy efforts up to 1966, only eleven major studies of effectiveness are noted by Wolf [7], and all have some serious defects in data or design. Possible relevant influence of family background and environment, supportive social and mental health services, improved neonatal care, and medical follow-up are among variables which may contribute significantly to a more favorable outlook for the affected child and are yet to be clearly delineated.

Perhaps we are in a better position now than ever before to identify and study the multiple factors using current computer technology. Moreover, the general climate of increased interest in and awareness of early identification and intervention has resulted in a proliferation of programs involving considerable numbers of children. The sizable populations participating in treatment programs offer the possibility of meaningful numbers for statistical analysis and detailed study, including large-scale collaborative efforts. Still, seriously lacking are effective instruments and procedures to gather the necessary data and study designs to ensure replicable research in a field committed to clinical service and long-term care.

Finally, it is clear that current practice with very young children is evolving into new and perhaps broader pathways. The field has moved from initially late identification and a predominantly orthopedic surgery/bracing approach to very early identification and the application of individual therapy modalities to the young child. More recently, the general process of early educationally oriented intervention treatment has come to the fore. This type of program might or might not include one or more of the therapy approaches. Our task is made more difficult, therefore, because we must now be aware of these education or medical models and their respective or interrelated effects as instruments of change in the infant who is exposed to them. Early intervention with or without specific therapy modalities is now the accepted and widely practiced procedure for the child identified as having developmental delays and possible cerebral palsy. This broader approach will mandate the use of objective assessment instruments to enable analysis of medical and/or educational oriented intervention in relation to developmental change in these children.

It seems that in the past 20 years, we have gone from a single variable therapy emphasis to a multidimensional approach in a headlong fashion and find ourselves in a situation today not unlike it was 20 years ago, when there was a polarization between the advocates and the nonbelievers. History seems to be repeating itself. Once again, we are faced with the problem of having to find effective scientific means of validating the clinical activities which consume so much of our professional time, effort, and budget. The question today is, are we able to document both the effects of therapy and early intervention which is all around us?

ASSESSMENT PROCEDURES AND INSTRUMENTS

The first issue in studying the effects of therapy or intervention modalities concerns use of evaluation procedures which will provide appropriate information about development and change. As our understanding of underlying neurological deficit and relevant variables has become more sophisticated so have the instruments and approaches to data gathering.

Narrative Reports and Case Histories

The simplest evaluation procedure is the narrative case report which generally reviews the patient's condition before and subsequent to a therapy program. Carlson was among the earliest workers to use this method of reporting [8]. The general format includes review of function in relation to therapy and the ascribing of change to the treatment procedure itself without necessarily considering the effect of growth, or comparing to a normal or even similarly handicapped patient. The case report continues to be used, often to substantiate a specific therapy modality [9-11].

Functional Inventories and Evaluations of Activities of Daily Living

A variety of test instruments have been used to assess changes in functional ability, especially activities of daily living (ADL) in relation to therapy. Deaver was among the earliest to use an ADL test of function [12]. Brown expanded on Deaver's wrok and developed an Elementary Motor Skill Inventory for the young child, as well as a Daily Activity Inventory and Progress Record for older children [13]. These instruments were later modified for children with atypical movement [14], and for children with cerebral palsy in special classes [15].

Hoberman et al. found Brown's ADL Test inadequate for the preschool child and developed a Baby's Daily Activity Test. This was later modified into the Functional Development Motor Scale based on a comparison with the normal development scales of Gesell [16]. This was a prototype of several tests which attempt to assess function of the handicapped child in relation to a "normal" standard for age.

Ingram et al. developed a Cerebral Palsy Activity Record also primarily based on Gesell schedules. Assessment information enabled development of motor and social age quotients for children aged 4 weeks to 5 years [17]. Unfortunately, type and degree of neurological abnormality was not included for interpretation. Jones devised a developmental test and chart relating function to age using Gesell and other developmental components. This was especially scaled for cerebral palsy patients and provided for addition of serial data to monitor rate and type of change [18].

Anderson et al. also used a charting procedure to evaluate function and change in the areas of speech, hand use, balance, locomotion, and maturity [19]. Data enabled preparation of profile for the child aged 1 month to 4 years. Footh and Logan later devised a Preschool Functional Activity Test specifically for the child with central nervous system deficit. It was an attempt to move away from simple Gesell norms and emphasized ability to adapt effectively, such as independently using a wheelchair [20].

Skill Tests

Crosland revised skill charts originally used by Phelps to analyze movement and range of motion [21]. Data were related to physical therapy procedures for tasks of lower extremities and to occupational therapy for activities of trunk and upper extremities. The tests were not graded by age and did not consider the quality of function.

Miller et al. also used a Motor Development Test for upper extremity activity [22]. This was related to an occupational therapy program.

Motor Ability Tests

Johnson applied the Gesell standards to a Motor Age test of extremity motor ability of children from 4 months to 6 years, who were compared with the normal [23,24]. The Bobaths later designed the Test Chart of Motor Ability [25], which was the first instrument to assess *quality* of movement and extent of abnormal postures in various positions. It was based on a normal development sequence and tests quality of function and developmental level rather than merely providing a physical measure of ability to function. Semans adapted the Bobath chart by arranging items in ascending order of complexity relative to central nervous system maturation with a grading system for each test item. Serial test profiles were used for assessment of change in motor ability [26].

Other motor development scoring systems have been in wide use. Zausmer and Tower developed a motor ability test as part of the American Academy for Cerebral Palsy's assessment instrument [27]. Scherzer et al. used a Motor Development Evaluation form grading presence and quality of motor patterns in prone, supine, sitting, quadruped, knee standing, standing, and walking. Presence and quality of primitive and postural reflexes were also included [28].

Development Profiles

Broad-scope assessment procedures involving various parameters of maturation have been utilized less frequently. Koven and Rowe prepared a five-point scale as a measure of degree of involvement. This included psychological and ambulatory status, ADL, and verbal ability [29]. No standardization was used.

Doman et al. have used several instruments to record related aspects of development. These include the Developmental Mobility Scale [30], the Doman-Moran Graphic Summary [31], and the Developmental Profile [32]. The latter records neurological integration based on developmental stages of motor, sensation, language, auditory, and tactile competency.

Pattern Analysis

Milani-Comparetti developed a chart to record patterns of movement (motoscopic observations) of trunk and extremities using notation similar to that used for choreography [33]. The record is to be used in comparison with notations of normal patterns.

A variety of visual methods have also been developed for recording and analyzing movement and particularly gait. These include light patterns [34], electromyography [35], and electronic or computer recordings [36], among others.

Clinical Assessments

By far the most commonly used procedure is general clinical assessment without following a particular form, check list, or formal test instrument. This is similar to the individual case report but may have no specific outline or form of reporting. It is a regular procedure of evaluation and reevaluation practiced by therapists to update patient progress. It is also approached in almost as many diverse ways as there are therapists. Content is often not uniform even with the same therapist, in a given center, or even with the same patients in subsequent reports. Therefore, it is often virtually impossible to compare reports of an individual patient under treatment with a previous performance or to assess a relation with normal or similarly affected individuals.

There is a wide variety of approaches to recording information about patients. The focus may be narrow and involve motor skills alone or discrete ADL functioning. It may broaden to include specific interrelated variables, or generally consider the total development or function of a patient utilizing a narrative case history. Many problems arise from the variety and types of assessments being used.

Lack of uniformity in reporting and use of several different test instruments within a therapy department of a treatment agency often prevents meaningful analysis of change for a given patient. Comparing results with patients from other agencies is further confounded by different types and extent of data. As yet there seems to be little agreement on the type of reporting form and extent of information which should be included either in the basic initial therapy work-up or in subsequent periodic reevaluations. This may reflect the growth and maturation of this field. However, without some generally agreed standards for data to be included in evaluations, the goal of a rational approach to understanding objectively the effect of treatment and planning appropriate modification will remain illusory.

Many assessment instruments continue to be based upon the "normal" sequence of neuromotor development as set forth generally in the Gesell standards. A major inherent weakness is the simple transferral of data from such standards to the developmentally impaired child [37]. Comparison with the age-normal child, for example, does not provide an indication of rate and quality of change. It may place the patient at continued disadvantage because discrete areas of change often occur which have not yet become part of functional development. These would include more mature reflex behavior or improved range of motion which have not yet been incorporated into functional activities.

Finally, objective reporting is often difficult to achieve. In the service-oriented milieu, the therapist who has devoted much time, effort, and skill to a patient cannot be faulted for being biased in favor of definite improvement as a result of these efforts. Irrespective of the assessment procedure, form, or test instrument used, if the observations are made by the treating therapist it is likely that such bias will affect the data to some extent. This may be further exaggerated by personality, and special interests of the therapist as well as program and budget considerations of the agency, among many possible factors.

SURVEY OF THERAPY STUDIES

An appropriate instrument to gauge the status of a child's development is a necessary and first condition in assessing individual progress and facilitating future treatment planning. That we are still far short of achieving this goal is amply demonstrated by the multitude of tests and procedures in current use, with their limitations.

Research on both effectiveness and value of the therapy intervention approach itself is beginning to develop with some degree of scientific sophistication. A major limitation in the past has been inadequacy of available patient information, a direct result of previously discussed problems relating to test instruments and assessment procedures. In addition, studies of treatment have generally not had a specific design, but instead merely reported patient data from a particular form of therapy. Until relatively recently no consideration has been given to identification of variables other than treatment which could influence development. The influence of physiological growth alone has still not been adequately studied, although control data are now more commonly utilized, and long-term effects of treatment are being more systematically considered. These are but a few of the continuing concerns arising from weakness of study design and present an impediment to progress within this field. Samples of the types of study designs currently in use are reviewed below.

Narrative Case Reviews

Individual case histories and narrative case reports have already been considered as patient assessment instruments. Much of the "research" up to the present still consists of such individual reports, often intending to substantiate one or another form of therapy. In some instances, these records have been brought together for numbers of patients to form a case review series. The individual clinical report serves as the data gathering method in a study design of case summaries. Information about outcome relates to motor development and functional ability.

Paine presented a classic case review follow-up study comparing "treated" with totally untreated patients known from 1930 to 1950 [38]. "Treatment" varied widely, was not consistent, and could not necessarily be well-documented, but was instituted in every instance at a relatively late age. Moreover, outcomes in neither treated nor untreated groups could be related to any of several possible associated variables such as age, intelligence, or degree of involvement. Under these circumstances it is not surprising that "treatment" seemed to make little difference for ambulation of the mild spastic hemiplegia patient on the one hand or for the severely involved athe-toid patient on the other. Similarly, no specific effect of therapy was seen among those who had undergone orthopedic surgery.

Clinical case reviews of patients receiving specific treatment procedures in-clude the early work of Kong [39]. Patients on Bobath treatment underwent repeat clinical evaluations after one to four years of therapy. Degree of in-volvement without indication of specific cerebral palsy diagnosis provided the basis for comparison. Satisfactory gait and minimal neurological signs were reported for this group. Woods did a similar clinical review of Bobath-treated patients and found a poorer prognosis for those with athetosis [40], but over-all significant improvement in functional and neurological status.

Treatment Studies with Specific Assessment Instruments

Crosland reported the first study of treatment results with nonspecific ther-apy methods using *skill tests* [21]. No analysis was available of relevant vari-ables. Both spastic and athetoid patients were reported to improve equally, and intelligence did not seem to be related to progress. Conflicting results were reported by Johnson using the *Motor Age Test* [24]. Here the data showed spastics responding better than athetoids; a higher IQ predicted better improvement; and many were thought to do as well without therapy. More responsive status for the spastic patient was again disputed by Ingram et al. using the *Cerebral Palsy Activity Record*. Patients were evaluated following intensive physical and occupational therapy.

Doman used a Mobility Scale to evaluate movement in children with mixed motor deficits receiving patterning treatment [30]. Encouraging re-sults were noted. Again, no analysis of possible associated influencing factors is given, nor is there mention of possible effect of growth and maturation alone. Similar studies of this method using the expanded *Doman-Delacato Profile* of general function indicate improved rates of neurological growth [31,32]. However, analysis of patient background and environmental fac-tors, among many other variables, is not available as in the initial study.

Adding to the inconsistent and often conflicting results with this group of studies is the work of Footh and Logan using the *PreSchool Functional Ac-tivities Test* [20]. They found no relationship to either previous or present physical therapy and no bearing of the IQ level on the effect of therapy.

Assessment of Management and Treatment

Finally, Carlsen compared results of two occupational therapy procedures in a small group of young children with cerebral palsy using perceptual and functional assessment evaluations (facilitation techniques vs. functional skill training) [41]. Definite improved developmental levels were noted as a result of this early intervention, particularly in the facilitation group.

Control Studies

Data from clinical evaluations, case reports, or the use of test instruments, leave undecided the question of placebo effect, or the role of growth alone, personality variables of the therapist, effect of the therapy visit itself, and many other possible confusing and conflicting factors which may color or influence any treatment regime. A research design which might resolve these concerns involves the use of controls. In this standard study design procedure, two comparable populations are identified. One receives the treatment procedure while the other serves as a control (untreated) group. Obviously, the closer the groups are matched, the more valid the comparison. Also, validity is enhanced if it is possible to mask the identity of treatment and control groups by physical separation, and appear to do similar things to both groups. This can be done by administering a "sham" procedure or similar device to the control group.

The control study design approach clearly offers many advantages in singling out the effect of the therapy procedure as the variable most directly related to change. However, much depends on the validity of the assessment instruments, comparability of the groups being compared, elimination of observor bias and other possible influencing factors.

This classic approach has been the hallmark of scientific research into many areas of related medical fields. The need for such studies is readily apparent in the cerebral palsy treatment area. Research of this design concerning established treatment modalities has just been emerging over the last several years concerning established treatment modalities.

Wright and Nicholson were among the first to attempt a prospective study on a group receiving a general physical therapy program [42]. Using a pre-post design with random assignment to groups, they felt improved function related to the therapy carryover and improved handling by parents. No significant difference was found between experimental and control groups.

Scherzer et al. used a double-blind research design to study the effect of physical therapy on cerebral palsy children under 18 months of age [28]. The treatment group received a combination of several presently accepted modalities of neurodevelopmental physical therapy; the control group utilized traditional passive range of motion exercises only. Assignment to groups was by random selection. Group matching was not attempted due to small sample size. Evaluating therapists and physicians were unaware of group assignments. A motor assessment instrument previously described was used to determine changes in motor status. Social change was determined through the Vineland Social Maturity Scale. Effect on home management was evaluated through pre- and posttest questionnaires completed by patients' families. In each of these areas the treatment group showed significant improvement.

Hochleitner then studied comparable groups of cerebral palsy patients with and without Bobath therapy [43]. No specific test instruments are described. Direct matching of the two groups was also not attempted. Cerebral palsy diagnoses varied as did severity and associated disabilities. Results of long-term follow-up show significant reduction in disability among the treatment group while controls continued with severe deficit. The initial severity of both groups is not given and could be a factor in later results if those who were initially more involved fell into the nontreated category. Nevertheless, those subjected to therapy clearly had significantly less residual disability when reevaluated.

Several subsequent studies with an experimental-control design are of interest. Goodman et al. [44] and Piper and Pless [45] dealt with infants at neurodevelopmental risk but without a specific diagnosis of cerebral palsy. In neither case were the treatment procedures found to be of significance in the outcome of subsequent development.

Reflecting the current shift in emphasis from a medical/therapy model of treatment to a more educationally oriented early intervention emphasis, Palmer et al. studied a group of infants with spastic diplegia [46].

They compared a randomly assigned group receiving neurodevelopmental physical therapy for 12 months to a group assigned to 6 months of educationally based infant stimulation program followed by 6 months of physical therapy. Blinded outcome assessment was undertaken after 6 and 12 months of therapy. On the questionable and selected outcome measures of incidence of contractures or need for bracing or orthopedic surgery, no significant difference was found for the study groups. On the contrary, the group receiving infant stimulation seemed to have done better on psychological testing (short-term) and overall motor development. While this study was based on a random design, its validity would have been considerably enhanced by the use of a control group not receiving either of the assigned modalities, and follow up assessment on a long-term basis. Other methodological weaknesses have previously been discussed in detail [47].

Other Studies

Rembolt developed an extensive compendium of past research in recent years in the categories described, with the exception of control studies [48].

An explosion of treatment investigation parallels the current trend toward early intervention in all types of developmental disabilities, often in young infants of whom a definitive neurological label cannot be placed [49]. Also more sophisticated control designs are now replacing case studies and narrative reviews [50] and computerization of data is enabling greater precision of multivariate analysis [51].

For example, utilizing the technique of meta analysis on 74 studies of early intervention programs, the University of Utah Early Intervention Research Institute found clearcut positive, developmental outcomes for the populations subjected to the programs, particularly for those who had longer exposure. Of some interest is the fact that there was less support found for the notion that those who had started at an earlier age, had a better outcome [52].

Meta analysis techniques represent increasing attempts to quantify and pool the results of large numbers of studies but have many limitations due to inherent weakness of individual data especially with comparability [53].

Finally, the single subject research design is being introduced as an effective means to assess developmental change over time in a given individual [54]. Particularly in situations where matched control studies are difficult to implement this method has specific advantages. However, it suffers from much less ability to generalize conclusions than in the control study design.

Status of Cerebral Palsy Research

The multihandicapping nature of cerebral palsy accentuates the problems of identifying both discrete and interrelated areas of development responding to treatment. Change occurs slowly and simultaneously with parallel growth and maturation. Identification and objective measurement of specific aspects of the child's functioning remain elusive but are necessary first steps in any meaningful study. The data are "soft" because quantitative measurement is generally not possible. One must resort to semiquantitative scales and descriptive profiles derived from many units of information.

Current evidence on the effect of early treatment in cerebral palsy is still weak but thought provoking, with clear trends confirming its validity. The evidence remains "soft." Sampling size has been insufficient in reports from many different geographical and environmental backgrounds. Comparability has not been possible due to lack of standardization in treatment procedures, types of evaluations, or reporting. Bias in sampling and evaluation remains the rule.

Often samples are small and heterogeneous, there is nonrandom assignment of treatment, limited use of control design, and followup is poor [53].

Too little attention has been given to objective recording in evaluations. Use of varied methods of data gathering such as questionnaires, interviews, and physiologic measurements has been frequently neglected as a variable. Only recently has study design itself been emphasized. Fortunately, considerable impetus for improvement is now coming from the work in developmental psychology and early intervention studies of the developmentally delayed child. There is now also an increasing sophistication in approaching such studies with a definite research design rather than a descriptive analysis of clinical experience alone.

A word must be said about parental expectation and evaluation. However the professionals may view the effect of a given therapy in general or in a particular child, at any point the parent will view developmental change in relation to preset goals and expectations of the therapy procedure. The value of treatment is still more extolled than proven and often turns on the convictions and personality of the therapist. Both may vary and change with individuals and as yet the parent must pursue through faith rather than hard data. This is the challenge for those whose clinical experience has confirmed the value of early treatment approach described in Chapters 4 to 9.

DEVELOPING EFFECTIVE STUDY DESIGNS

Review of current studies has shown some encouraging trends in effecting de-development changes through early intervention therapy, be it specific physical therapy or a more educationally oriented approach. Validity of the data remains in question, however, because of weaknesses in the quality and objectivity of information, the inability as yet of totally excluding interference from other possible factors which may cause change, and designs which do not fully enable comparison with those left untreated. That these conditions continue in spite of highly sophisticated research efforts in today's behavioral sciences and related "soft data" fields is a reflection of the special circumstance of this service-oriented field. The problem of demonstrating irrefutable evidence that early therapy makes a significant difference remains, even after years of treatment efforts. This base must first be fully established. Having done so, the next and persistent challenge will be to determine which types of therapy and special conditions are most appropriate for a particular child with specific deficits, that is the search for a discrete prescriptive approach to treatment based on known effect and long-term follow-up. These goals may, in fact be attainable if we can understand better the special conditions, problems, and obstacles which are likely to affect any research effort in this field.

Research Obstacles

THERAPISTS IN THE RESEARCH MILIEU

Therapy is committed to servicing and treating those in need. It is an action-oriented profession. As in any clinical setting, the *personality of the therapist* may have a major bearing on the response of the patient, *no matter which procedure is being followed.* From the very beginning, therefore, an element of influence may be introduced whose effect could be crucial. This is a variable which will have to be anticipated and "controlled" or at least recognized in any study of treatment results.

Because therapists are caring individuals and may be closely associated with a particular type or school of therapy, they are often convinced that their treatment will work and will be beneficial to patients even before starting. This is especially and increasingly true today as many centers are exclusively providing a particular form of treatment such as neurodevelopmental therapy (NDT).

The therapy program is often viewed by the therapist as a unique and specific treatment in itself, comparable to a dose of medication. Often it is not placed in the perspective of an approach requiring practice and carryover at home or a direction for behavioral stimulation, which is generally regarded as its basis of operation. To withhold treatment from some or to modify conditions to enable study is for many therapists at best a rejection of their perceived role and at worst a deception of the patient or family. No wonder the therapist often objects to studies in which there is selection and control of patients or where the conditions require some alteration from the accustomed treatment regime.

Finally, the therapist often develops a unique rapport with the family and is the major avenue of communication for anything which influences the child. A perceived alteration in treatment required for study purposes or a negative response by the therapist to a study procedure, could be quickly recognized by the parent and affect much-needed cooperation.

The focal role of the therapist as an influential committed individual must be fully delineated and respected. When this issue is fully understood it will be possible to utilize the inherent strengths of therapy staff to help design and participate in more objective approaches to understanding the effects of treatment.

The early introduction of educational models of treatment further complicates professional bias by bringing together those with a somewhat different orientation and background. It means that both therapists and teaching staff must communicate well and respect each other's disciplines in order to develop the most effective program and ultimately allow for its objective evaluation.

CONTROLLING ENVIRONMENTAL AND OTHER INFLUENCES

The therapist/teacher is one of several major variables which may affect developmental change. Home conditions, interest, adjustment and response of family members, particularly in providing stimulation, and in expectations, are also among the most potentially relevant. An accurate picture of these factors is essential so that their possible or potential effect on the child's development can be assessed in relation to the treatment procedure and results.

SAMPLING

A major problem is that frequently only small numbers of children are under treatment in a given center or program. This may be a reflection of a relatively small infant population in some areas or limited referrals of very young children with suspected early developmental deficits. The latter continues to be a major problem stemming from limited awareness of early identification by practitioners and/or lack of conviction of the value of early intervention. The sample size will therefore often not enable matching, comparing, control designs, or other means of statistical design. It is also often not possible to deal with narrow ranges of homogeneous age, diagnosis, or degree of disability ranges, and instead more heterogeneous groupings must be used. This reduces the ability to deal specifically with unique groupings and the resulting data often becomes far too general.

A possible solution to this problem is the organization of large-scale collaborative studies. Comparable groups are identified in multiple centers, each receiving identical interventions under conditions which are comparably controlled. By this means, sufficiently large numbers of subjects under investigation enable use of sophisticated statistical techniques. This procedure is already well-established in several areas of medical care including treatment of renal disease [55], leukemia [56], and in the previous collaborative maternal and infant study of cerebral palsy etiology [57].

SELECTING AND USING TESTING INSTRUMENTS

Much has already been said about the problems in collecting data and information relating to developmental change. Uniformity is the greatest need in developing initial and follow-up evaluations so that records are complete and comparable. The assessment instrument to be used is often selected on the basis of "normal" developmental standards and frequently does not allow an adequate understanding of rate of change for a given individual irrespective of chronological expectations. Also assessments may depend heavily on only the clinical judgment of the evaluating professional without specific objective measurement guidelines.

RECORDING AND INTERPRETING DATA

Observer bias is the single most difficult research obstacle with which to deal. Often therapists are convinced that their prescribed treatment is most effective with no need for an alternative approach. A possible solution is to use another therapist to perform reevaluations in a masked fashion, and record and interpret the data regarding developmental change. This could have many obvious advantages, not the least of which is to encourage more objective reporting.

USE OF CONTROLS

Many of the studies reported have an inherent design of comparing the patient with his or her previous level of development and function. This is a well-established procedure in which the individual serves as his or her own control [58]. While this method gives the appearance of an effective objective procedure, it has some definite weaknesses. First, in the time since the initial or previous evaluation, numerous factors other than the treatment procedure itself could be operative in effecting change. These might include changes in environmental conditions, such as parental interest or support, physical developmental acceleration, or the addition of other environmental stimulation not previously available. Clearly, it must be specifically ascertained that, during the periods being compared, changed conditions or other possible influencing variables can be discounted.

Actual matched control studies of early intervention therapy are just now beginning to emerge, as previously discussed. The limitations relate to frequent small sample size which prevents effective matching, resistance by therapists and other staff to withholding any treatment from young children for the sake of research, and the ever-present difficulties of selection of appropriate assessment instruments and reducing bias in reporting. Each of these can be dealt with if the involved professional is aware of the implications of his or her role and can grasp the advantages of achieving reputable research findings to substantiate the place of therapy in affecting development of infants with neurological deficit.

Planning for Effective Patient Assessments

The following is a suggested guide to the clinical approach to patient assessments. The need for reasonable completeness, uniformity, consistency, and objectivity pervades all facets of the evaluation of patients. The extent to which these guidelines are followed will determine potential for accurate long-term follow of individual patients as well as ultimate comparability among groups of children being treated at numerous centers.

INITIAL EVALUATION

1. Schedule adequate time for a full evaluation schedule to meet the specific goals of the therapy program.
2. Provide an appropriate, reasonably quiet place where interruption will be minimized.
3. Predetermine specific areas of development to be assessed: consider confining evaluation to one or more of the following:
   a. Motor development—baseline assessment including:
      i. Assessment of tone and reflex behavior
      ii. Limitations in range of motion
      iii. Review base of support in any position
      iv. Assess center of gravity over base of support
   b. Functional ability—ADL
   c. Social maturation—management level
   d. Oral development/speech.
4. Prepare assessment form in outline, if possible, with check-off design.
5. Summarize findings, short- and long-range therapy goals, and plan of treatment.
6. Plan in advance for schedule of reevaluation assessments.
7. Review plans with other therapies/teachers for gaps and overlap in treatment. The combined effect is to prepare for each child an Individual Development Plan (IDP).

REEVALUATIONS

1. Set aside regularly scheduled periods in quiet conditions for reevaluations.
2. Develop a suitable reevaluation form in check-off style, if possible, for each developmental area being considered (see appendix).
3. Summarize findings: prepare new short- and long-range goals, revising previous plans as appropriate.
4. Maintain regular schedule of reevaluations using prepared forms. Suggested intervals would be more frequent with very young children (about every three months), and less often as the child grows. Examinations should be at least twice annually.
5. Continue regular joint reevaluations with entire therapy team for full review and planning.

The goal is for all therapists/teachers to develop an appreciation of the objective and thorough evaluation process as a major integral professional responsibility. Without question this is on a par with actual physical contact and treatment of the child.

Guidelines for Therapy Research

Adequate clinical assesments, instruments, and procedures are a first requirement in developing objective information on the child's level of development and function. Only after these are developed can study be initiated on the effects of a particular therapy or intervention modality. While pactitioners must be aware of the obstacles and difficulties inherent in research in this area, the following guidelines are offered for those who have an interest in planning research or better interpreting and understanding research reports:

1. Gain the interest, confidence and acceptance of staff through frank discussion of the need and purposes of research studies.
2. Begin any study with an objective outlook toward the benefit of a treatment procedure.
3. Develop a design which will avoid or eliminate possible interfering environmental influence and other spurious variables.
4. Consider the use of control designs with matching of samples if possible.
5. Use a large enough sample to develop the data properly. Consider possible data sharing and collaboration with other comparable centers. Use objective random or other statistically valid sampling techniques.
6. Select assessment instructions for objectivity, completeness and relevance to research goals.
7. Utilize objective therapist/teacher evaluations by nontreating (masked) therapists where possible.
8. Obtain results of parent, teacher, and other relevant professionals' interviews and questionnaires both prior to and during therapy to develop information about expectations and outcomes.
9. Be consistent in following out the research design with proper sampling assessments and objective recording of data until required sample number is complete.

While no single set of guidelines will assure quality of research, it is clear that a well-prepared and executed design is the best hope for a meaningful study. This is clearly a major need in the therapy field and could do much to strengthen standards for treatment and professional growth. A solid research foundation is the necessary ingredient to firmly establish the relevance of both early evaluation and infant intervention programs.

THERAPY IN WORLD PERSPECTIVE

Broader and perhaps more sophisticated dimensions of concern now face us as well. America and the western industrial nations have had the resources and technological capability to develop what is considered to be the "standard" of treatment in this field. This is the case even though we continue to lack adequate scientific validity of our methods, as we have seen. At any rate, we have until recently applied our procedures as best we can *primarily* within our own societies and cultures.

We can now begin to see some extension in the application of our technology beyond our own borders. For a new revolutionary component is upon us. In spite of ever-present infectious diseases and malnutrition, increasing numbers of children are now surviving with greater frequency. According to United Nations estimates, some two thirds of the world's 500 million handicapped children live in the Third World nations alone [59].

A number of official agencies such as UNICEF/WHO, individual governments, and nongovernmental organizations, are now actively involved in working with these areas on problems with the handicapped. Confusion, overlapping, and duplication in efforts seem to be a mark of these activities, largely due to the numbers of agencies and programs involved, as well as problems in communication and information exchange between them.

More important, the direct application of our purely Western technology and methods is obviously impractical economically, and clearly inappropriate culturally. Both WHO and UNICEF have recently recognized the need to overcome these obstacles and have helped initiate the community-based rehabilitation movement [60]. In Sri Lanka [61], the Philippines [62], Jamaica [63], Botswana and Zimbabwe [64], and a number of other Third World countries, projects have begun at the grass roots level, often initiated locally. Technical personnel train local individuals in rudimentary early identification of handicaps, simple methods of treatment, and use of local materials for needed equipment. This type of activity will surely be in greater demand as we can anticipate an increasing population of the handicapped in these areas with little likelihood for improved resources in the foreseeable future. Indeed, a sizable literature is emerging on self-help activities at the grass roots level [66].

The time has come for us, therefore, to begin to use our expertise to assist in this effort. We need to have a firmer grasp on the relevance of our own therapy and treatment methods, through the kinds of studies we have previously indicated. We must then have the skill and wisdom in adapting them to cultures elsewhere, such as the Third World, where there is need for a simple, economically feasible, and practical approach [66]. Any system of therapy which has evolved, will have little relevance unless it takes into account the social and cultural context of a disability, rather than simply the diagnosis alone. It is time for us all to have this kind of world perspective in our treatment efforts.

REFERENCES

1. Green, W., and McDermott, L. Operative treatment of cerebral palsy of the spastic type. *JAMA* 118:434, 1942.

2. Couch, W., De Rosa, G., and Throop, F. Thigh adductor transfer for spastic cerebral palsy. *Dev. Med. Child Neurol.* 19:343, 1977.

3. Louick, D., and Boland, T. Psychologic tests: A guide for pediatricians. *Pediatr. Ann.* 7:86, 1978.

4. Barrera, M., et al. Early intervention with biologically handicapped infants and young children: A preliminary study with each child as his own control. In Tjossem, T. (ed): Intervention Strategies for High Risk Infants and Young Children. Baltimore, University Park Press, 1976, pp. 609-627.

5. Hayden, A., and Haring, N. Early intervention for high risk infants and young children: Programs for Down's syndrome children. In Tjossem, T. (ed): Intervention Strategies for High Risk Infants and Young Children. Baltimore, University Park Press, 1976, pp. 573-607.

6. Aronson, M., and Fallstrom, K. Immediate and long-term effects of developmental training in children with Down's syndrome. *Dev. Med. Child Neurol.* 19:489, 1977.

7. Wolf, J. The Results of Treatment in Cerebral Palsy. Springfield, Charles C Thomas, 1969.

8. Carlson, E. Motor re-eeducation in birth injuries—a case report. *Yale J. Biol. Med.* 3:49, 1940-1931.

9. Wainer, G. Psychotherapy in a girl of 18 years with severe cerebral palsy. *Dev. Med. Child Neurol.* 7:175, 1965.

10. Spira, R. Management of spasticity in cerebral palsied children by peripheral nerve block with phenol. *Dev. Med. Child Neurol.* 13:164, 1971.

11. Skrotzky, K., Gallenstein, J., and Osternig, L. Effects of electromyographic feedback training on motor control in spastic cerebral palsy. *Phys. Ther.* 58:547, 1978.

12. Deaver, G., and Brown, M. Physical Demands of Daily Life. Studies in Rehabilitation No. 1. New York. Institute for Crippled and Disabled, 1945.

13. Brown, M. Daily activity testing and teaching. *Phys. Ther. Rev.* 27:249, 1947.

14. Brown, M. Daily activity inventory and progress record for those with atypical movement. *Am. J. Occup. Ther.* 4:195, 1950.

15. Brown, M. Daily activity inventories of cerebral palsied children in experimental classes. *Phys. Ther. Rev.* 20:415, 1950.

16. Hoberman, M., Cicenia, E., and Stephenson, C. A useful measurement tool in the physical rehabilitation program of pre-school orthopedically handicapped children. *Arch. Phys. Med.* 32:457, 1951.

17. Ingram, A., Withers, E., and Spetz, E. Role of intensive physical and occupational therapy in the treatment of cerebral palsy: Testing and results. *Arch. Phys. Med.* 40:429, 1959.

18. Jones, M. Appraisal of Progress in the Cerebral Palsied Child. Los Angeles, United Cerebral Palsy of Los Angeles County, 1952.

19. Anderson, R., Bargowski, E., and Blodgett, W. A Code Method for Evaluating Function in Cerebral Palsy. Detroit Orthopedic Clinic, 1961.

20. Footh, V., and Logan, K. Measuring the effectiveness of physical therapy in the treatment of cerebral palsy. *J. Am. Phys. Ther. Assoc.* 43:867, 1967.

21. Crosland, J. The assessment of results in the conservative treatment of cerebral palsy. *Arch. Dis. Child.* 26:92, 1951.

22. Miller, A., Stewart, M., Murphy, M., and Jantzin, A. An evaluation method for cerebral palsy. *Am. J. Occup. Ther.* 9:105, 1955.

23. Johnson, M., Zuck, F., and Wingate, K. The Motor Age Test: measurement of motor handicaps in children with neuromuscular disorders such as cerebral palsy. *J. Bone Joint Surg.* [Am] 33:698, 1951.

24. Johnson, M. The use of the Motor Age Test in the evaluation of cerebral palsy patients. *Instruct. Lect. Am. Acad. Orthop. Surg.* 9:108, 1952.

25. Bobath, K., and Bobath, B. An assessment of the motor handicap of

children with cerebral palsy and their response to treatment. *Am. J. Occup. Ther.* 2:19, 1958.

26. Semans, S. A cerebral palsy assessment chart. *J. Am. Phys. Assoc.* 45: 463, 1965.

27. Zausmer, E., and Tower, G. A quotient for the evaluation of motor development. *J. Am. Phys. Ther. Assoc.* 46:725, 1966.

28. Scherzer, A., Mike, V., and Ilson, J. Physical therapy as a determinant of change in the cerebral palsied infant. *Pediatrics* 58:47, 1976.

29. Koven, L, and Rowe, R. A general capacities scale for children with neuromotor handicaps. *Am. J. Occup. Ther.* 13:166, 1959.

30. Doman, G., Delacato, C., and Doman, R. The Doman-Delacato Developmental Mobility Scale. Philadelphia, The Rehabilitation Center, 1960.

31. Doman, G., and Moran, P. The Doman-Moran Graphic Summary. Philadelphia, The Institutes for the Achievement of Human Potential, 1963.

32. Doman, G., Delacato, C., and Doman, R. The Doman-Delacato Developmental Profile. Philadelphia, The Rehabilitation Center, 1962.

33. Milani-Comparetti, A., and Gidoni, E. Pattern analysis of motor development and its disorders. *Dev. Med. Child Neurol.* 9:625, 1967.

34. Aptekar, R., Ford, F., and Bleck, E. Light patterns as a means of assessing and recording gait. II results in children with cerebral palsy. *Dev. Med. Child Neurol.* 18:37, 1976.

35. Csongradi, J., Bleck, E., and Ford, F. Gait electromyography in normal and spastic children, with special reference to quadriceps femoris and hamstring muscles. *Dev. Med. Child Neurol.* 21:738, 1979.

36. Close, J. Motor Function in the Lower Extremity. Analyses by Electronic Instrumentation. Springfield, Charles C Thomas, 1964.

37. Semans, S. Specific tests and evaluation tools for the child with central nervous system deficit. *J. Am. Phys. Ther. Assoc.* 45:457, 1965.

38. Paine, R. On the treatment of cerebral palsy: The outcome of 177 patients, 74 totally untreated. *Pediatrics* 29:605, 1962.

39. Kong, E. Very early treatment of cerebral palsy. *Dev. Med. Child Neurol.* 9:198, 1966.

40. Woods, G. The outcome of physical treatment in cerebral palsy. *Cerebral Palsy Rev.* 25:3, 1964.

41. Carlsen, P. Comparison of two occupational therapy approaches for treating the young cerebral palsied child. *Am. J. Occup. Ther.* 29:267, 1975.

42. Wright, T., and Nicholson, J. Physiotherapy for the spastic child—an evaluation. *Dev. Med. Child Neurol.* 15:146,1973.

43. Hochleitner, M. Vergleichende Untersuchung von Kindern mit zerebraler Bewegungsstörung, mit under ohne neuro-physiologischer Fruhtherapie. *Oestr. Aerzt.* 32:1108, 1977.

44. Goodman, M., Rothberg, A., Houston-McMillan, J., et al. Effect of early neurodevelopmental therapy in normal and at risk survivors of neonatal intensive care. *Lancet* II:1327, 1985.

45. Piper, M., and Pless, I. Early intervention for infants with Down syndrome: A controlled trial. *Pediatrics* 65:465, 1980.

46. Palmer, F., Shapiro, B., Wachtel, R., Allen, R., et al. The effects of physical therapy on cerebral palsy: a controlled trial in infants with spastic diplegia. *N. Engl. J. Med.* 318:803, 1988.

47. Bax, M. Controlled trial of physical therapy at Johns Hopkins. Editorial. *Dev. Med. Child Neurol.* 30:285, 1988.

48. Rembolt, R., and Roth, B. (eds.). Cerebral Palsy and Related Developmental Disabilities—Prevention and Early Care. An annotated Bibliography, Vols. I-III. Columbus, Ohio State University Press, 1975.

49. Tjossem, T. (ed). Intervention Strategies for the High Risk Infant. Baltimore, University Park Press, 1976.

50. Leib, S., Benfiedl, G., and Guidubaidi, J. Effects of early intervention and stimulation of the pre-term infant. *Pediatrics* 66:83, 1980.

51. Zar, J. Biostatistical Analysis. Englewood Cliffs, NJ, Prentice-Hall, 1974, p. 190.

52. Castro, G., and Mastropieri, M. The efficacy of early intervention programs: A meta analysis. *Excep. Child.* 52:417, 1986.

53. Ottenbacher, K., and Peterson, P. The efficacy of early intervention programs for children with organic impairment: a quantitative review. *Eval. Progr. Plan.* 8:135, 1985.

54. Harris, S. Early intervention: does developmental therapy make a difference? *Topics Early Child. Spec. Educ.* 7:20, 1988.

55. Spitzer, A. et al. Prospective controlled trial of cyclophosphamide ther-

apy in children with nephrotic syndrome. A Report for the Information Study of Kidney Disease in Children. *Lancet* 2:423, 1974.

56. Miller, D. Prognostic factors in childhood acute lymphoblastic leukemia. *J. Pediatr.* 87:672, 1974.

57. Nelson, K., and Ellenberg, J. Neonatal signs as predictors of cerebral palsy. *Pediatrics* 64:225, 1979.

58. Martin, J., and Epstein, L. Evaluating treatment effectiveness in cerebral palsy: single-subject designs. *Phys. Ther.* 56:285, 1976.

59. Hammerman, S., and Irwin, M. (Eds.). Community based rehabilitation: essence of the new strategy in childhood rehabilitation. *UNICEF/RI One in Ten* 1:1, 1981.

60. Helander, E., Mendis, P., and Nelson, G. Training Disabled People in the Community—A Manual on Community Based Rehabilitation for Developing Countries. Geneva, WHO, 1983.

61. Kgosana, P. Within reach and yet beyond reach—a project for the prevention and control of childhood disabilities in Anuradhapura Town, Sri Lanka. Urban Examples for Basic Services Development in Cities. *UNICEF, UE* 11:29, 1985.

62. Periquet, A. Community Based Rehabilitation Services: The Experience of Bacolod, Philippines and the Asia—Pacific Region. New York, World Rehabilitation Fund, 1984.

63. McINtosh, S. Something positive to offer! *UNICEF News* 105:12, 1980.

64. Hammerman, S., and Habibi, G. (Eds.). Red Cross programs in community based rehabilitation in Botswana and Zimbabwe. *UNICEF/RI One in Ten* 3:4, 1984.

65. Werner, D. *Disabled Village Children—A Guide for Community Health Workers, Rehabilitation Workers and Families.* Palo Alto, Hesperian Foundation, 1987.

66. Scherzer, A. Guest Editorial: Toward a world perspective. *Dev. Med. Child Neurol.* 28:557, 1986.

APPENDIX Reevaluation

Name: Chart No.: Birth Date: Date: Therapist:

Date of Last Report:

I. Summary of Last Report:

II. Program Goals of Last Report:

III. Changes of Behavior as Compared with Last Report
    1. Functional Abilities:

    2. Motor Patterns
        Normal Postural Adaptations (Righting reactions, head control, postural symmetry and midline control, shoulder girdle stability, trunk control and proximal stability, protective extension of the arms, equilibrium reactions, manipulation and eye–hand–foot coordination, differentiation and variability of movements):

        Abnormal Postural Responses (exaggerated tonic reflexes, predominant hyperextension of head and neck, predominant scapular protraction/retraction, total and ungraded extensor patterns, pronounced/compensatory flexion, pronounced anterior/posterior pelvic tilt, stereotyped behavior, paucity/excess of movements):

APPENDIX Reevaluation (continued)

Postural Tonus (normal, hypotonic, hypertonic, rigid, fluctuating, associated reactions)
At rest:
Changes in response to stimulation, handling, movement:

3. Overall Quality of Motor Behavior (variability, grading, sequencing):

4. Predominant Motor Patterns:

5. Restricted Mobility, (Risk for) Contractures, Deformities:

6. Reaction to Sensory Stimulation (kinesthetic, tactile, auditory, visual):

IV. Additional Comments:

V. Summary:

VI. Program Goals:

VII. Recommended Procedures:

Index

About the Authors

ALFRED L. SCHERZER is Clinical Professor of Pediatrics and Adjunct
Professor of Public Health at Cornell University Medical College, New York
City, and Clinical Professor of Preventive Medicine at the State University
of New York School of Medicine, Stony Brook. He also serves as Director
of Pediatric Habilitation, New York Hospital; Director of the Child Habili-
tation Center, Central Suffolk Hospital, Long Island, New York; Senior
Medical Consultant to the United Cerebral Palsy Association of New York
City; and Medical Consultant to the New York City Board of Education,
Division of Special Education, and the Board of Cooperative Education
Services in eastern Long Island, New York. His research interests and writings reflect varied clinical experience in all pediatric handicapping conditions
and focus on long-term effects of treatment. Dr. Scherzer is the editor of
the Pediatric Habilitation series (Marcel Dekker, Inc.). He is a past president of the American Academy for Cerebral Palsy and Developmental Medicine, and current chairman of its International Affairs Committee. He received the M.S.P.H. (1950), Ed.D. (1954), and M.D. (1963) degrees from
Columbia University, New York City.

INGRID TSCHARNUTER is a Physical Therapist in private practice and a
Consultant to therapists and treatment programs in the New York Metro-
politan area. She also serves as an Adjunct Instructor of the advanced master's
degree program in developmental disabilities at New York University, New York
City, a frequent lecturer at conferences and seminars on developmental dis-

abilities and an instructor in N.D.T. (neuro-developmental treatment) certification courses and workshops throughout the U.S., Canada, and abroad. Ms. Tscharnuter is a member of the Neuro-Developmental Treatment Instructors' Group and an associate member of the American Academy for Cerebral Palsy and Developmental Medicine. She studied human development at the University of Vienna, Austria, and received the Phyiscal Therapist License (1964) from the School of Allied Health Professions in Vienna. Since that time she has examined various therapy approaches to developmental disorders throughout the world and worked in rehabilitation and pediatrics in Austria, Sweden, and the U.S. Ms. Tscharnuter was certified as N.D.T. (Bobath) therapist (1970) in Vienna and N.D.T. (Bobath) coordinator/instructor (1980) in the U.S.